BOOSTING LIFE BAR

Weaponizing Diet And Your Mindset For Healing

Introduction

The Power of Diet and Mindset in Healing

In a world where chronic inflammation has become an invisible epidemic, affecting everything from our joints to our digestive systems, our cardiovascular health to our emotional wellbeing, a revolution in healing is quietly taking place. This revolution isn't happening in pharmaceutical laboratories or hospital corridors, though those spaces remain vital. Instead, it's occurring in kitchens and consciousness—at the intersection of what we eat and how we think.

You've likely picked up this book because inflammation has touched your life in some way. Perhaps you're navigating the challenges of an autoimmune condition, struggling with digestive issues, experiencing the hormonal shifts of menopause, or simply feeling that your body isn't functioning as vibrantly as you know it could. Whatever brought you here, know this: you've taken a powerful step toward reclaiming your health.

The anti-inflammatory approach presented in these pages isn't a diet in the conventional sense—a temporary restriction to be endured before returning to old habits. Rather, it's a sustainable way of nourishing your body with foods that naturally combat inflammatory processes while avoiding those that trigger them. What makes this approach distinct, however, is its recognition that true healing requires more than just changing what's on your plate. It demands a transformation in how you relate to your body, your health challenges, and the healing process itself.

The Dual Path to Wellness

Chronic inflammation doesn't develop in isolation. It emerges from a complex interplay of factors: genetic predispositions, environmental triggers, lifestyle choices, and—critically—psychological states. Research increasingly confirms what traditional healing systems have long understood: the mind and body are not separate entities but aspects of an integrated whole, constantly communicating through an intricate network of neural pathways, hormones, and immune signals.

When we experience chronic stress, our bodies produce cortisol and other stress hormones that can trigger and perpetuate inflammatory responses. Negative thought patterns about our health can activate similar physiological pathways. Conversely, states of calm, compassion, and positive expectation create biochemical environments that support healing and reduce inflammation.

This book honors this profound mind-body connection by offering a comprehensive approach that addresses both nutritional and psychological dimensions of inflammation. You'll find not just recipes that soothe inflammatory pathways, but strategies for cultivating a mindset that supports your body's natural healing abilities.

Beyond Symptom Management

Conventional approaches to inflammatory conditions often focus exclusively on symptom management—suppressing pain, reducing visible inflammation, or controlling abnormal immune responses. While symptom relief is undeniably important, this approach alone rarely addresses the root causes of inflammation or supports the body's innate capacity for balance and regeneration.

The anti-inflammatory diet and mindset practices outlined in this book aim deeper. By providing your body with nutrients that modulate immune function, support cellular repair, and neutralize inflammatory compounds, while simultaneously cultivating thought patterns that reduce stress hormones and promote healing responses, you create conditions for comprehensive wellness—not just absence of symptoms.

This doesn't mean abandoning conventional medical treatments when needed. Rather, it means complementing them with natural approaches that address foundational aspects of health that medications alone cannot reach.

Weaponizing Hope For Healing

To you, the warrior facing health challenges on your journey—

Whether you're navigating the stormy waters of chronic inflammation, dancing with autoimmune conditions, weathering the changes of menopause, or simply seeking relief from persistent discomfort, I see your courage.

The path to healing often feels lonely. There are days when pain becomes your unwelcome companion, when fatigue drapes over you like a heavy blanket, when medical terms replace normal conversation, and when hope seems just beyond reach.

But within these pages lies a gentle truth: your body has an innate wisdom and capacity for healing. Food is not just sustenance—it is medicine, comfort, and a powerful ally in your quest for wellness.

This book is my hand extended to yours, offering not just recipes but possibilities. Each ingredient selected with purpose, each meal designed to reduce inflammation, support your immune system, and nurture your body's natural healing abilities.

Remember that healing is rarely linear. There will be good days and challenging ones. Progress might appear as subtle shifts—a night of better sleep, a morning with less stiffness, moments of clarity amid brain fog, or simply the joy of a delicious meal that loves your body back.

You are not defined by your diagnosis. Your worth is not measured by your productivity on difficult days. And you are never, ever alone in this journey.

As you turn these pages and bring these recipes to life in your kitchen, know that you're taking active steps toward reclaiming your health, one nourishing meal at a time. This is not just about eliminating inflammatory foods—it's about embracing a lifestyle that honors your body's needs and celebrates its remarkable resilience.

May this book serve as both practical guide and steadfast companion. May these recipes bring not only healing nutrients but also the simple pleasure of good food. And may you find, between these covers and within yourself, renewed hope and the quiet strength to continue forward.

To your health, your healing, and your wholeness,

With deep care and unwavering belief in your journey.

The Power of Mind: A Healing Journey

Sarah's Turning Point

Sarah winced as she lowered herself onto the edge of her bed, the familiar ache in her joints announcing itself like an unwelcome visitor. At 42, she'd been battling inflammatory arthritis for nearly five years, with her condition steadily worsening despite a carousel of medications. The constant pain had become her companion, dictating what she could do, where she could go, even how she thought about her future.

"This isn't living," she whispered to herself, tears threatening to spill. "It's just existing."

That night, unable to sleep, Sarah found herself scrolling through an online support group. One post caught her attention—a woman describing her journey with an anti-inflammatory diet coupled with mindfulness practices. The woman hadn't claimed a miracle cure, but rather a partnership: her mind and her nutrition working together to reduce inflammation and reclaim her life.

Something clicked for Sarah. She had tried various diets before, even attempted meditation, but always as separate strategies. What if they were two halves of the same healing approach?

The Mind-Body Connection

Dr. Elena Martinez, a rheumatologist specializing in integrative medicine, explains this connection: "Science increasingly shows us that chronic inflammation is influenced by both physical and psychological factors. Stress hormones like cortisol can actually trigger inflammatory responses, creating a cycle where physical inflammation and mental distress feed each other."

This understanding—that our thoughts and emotions aren't separate from our physical health but intricately connected to it—forms the foundation of what researchers call the psychoneuroimmunological approach to healing.

Michael's Battle with IBD

Michael had spent eight years with severe inflammatory bowel disease, his life revolving around bathroom locations and medication schedules. His gastroenterologist had suggested dietary changes, which helped somewhat, but breakthrough flares continued to disrupt his life.

During a particularly severe hospitalization, a nurse practitioner sat with him and asked an unexpected question: "How do you speak to yourself about your condition?"

Michael was taken aback. "What do you mean?"

"When you feel symptoms starting, what's your internal dialogue?"

Michael thought for a moment. "Usually panic. 'Oh no, not again.' 'I can't handle another flare.' 'Why is my body betraying me?'"

The nurse nodded. "That's completely understandable. But what if those thoughts themselves are part of the inflammatory cascade?"

She introduced Michael to a visualization practice where he imagined his immune system as an overeager guardian that needed gentle guidance rather than an enemy to be fought. Alongside continuing his anti-inflammatory nutrition plan, Michael began spending fifteen minutes each morning in this visualization, picturing healing, calm, and balance returning to his digestive system.

"It felt strange at first," Michael admits. "Almost like make-believe. But I had tried everything else. What did I have to lose?"

The Science of Mind Over Inflammation

The connection between mental state and inflammation isn't just anecdotal. Studies have shown that chronic stress can increase inflammatory markers in the blood, while mindfulness practices can reduce them. One landmark study at the University of Wisconsin-Madison found that mindfulness meditation could actually affect gene expression related to inflammation.

Dr. James Carson, who studies pain management at Oregon Health & Science University, explains: "When we change our relationship with pain through mindfulness, we're not just distracting ourselves—we're actually influencing the neurochemical processes that govern inflammation."

Emma's Migraine Relief

Emma had suffered debilitating migraines since her teens. By her thirties, she was experiencing 15-20 migraine days per month despite trying numerous medications. Her neurologist suggested an elimination diet to identify possible food triggers, which helped reduce frequency to about 10 episodes monthly—better, but still life-altering.

During a particularly hopeless period, Emma's friend gave her a book on neuroplasticity—the brain's ability to reorganize and form new neural connections. Intrigued, Emma began researching the relationship between thought patterns and pain perception.

"I realized I'd developed a fear-based relationship with my body," Emma explains. "I was constantly scanning for early migraine signs, living in dread of the next attack. That hypervigilance itself was creating stress, which ironically made migraines more likely."

Emma committed to combining her anti-inflammatory diet with two practices: gratitude journaling and progressive muscle relaxation. Each morning, she wrote down three things her body had done well. Each evening, she systematically relaxed each muscle group while visualizing healthy blood flow to her brain.

"Within two months, I was down to 4-5 migraines monthly," Emma shares. "After six months, just 1-2. The intensity decreased too. I still follow my nutrition plan religiously, but addressing the mind component was what finally broke the cycle."

The Power of Expectation

The placebo effect — where belief in a treatment creates real physiological improvement — demonstrates the remarkable power of expectation. But this effect isn't limited to sugar pills in clinical trials.

"Our expectations shape our biological responses in profound ways," explains neuroscientist Dr. Farah Khan. "When we genuinely believe healing is possible, our bodies release different chemicals than when we're convinced we'll remain sick. This isn't magical thinking — it's neurochemistry."

Robert, who struggled with psoriasis for decades, experienced this firsthand. After beginning an anti-inflammatory regimen, he added a daily affirmation practice, repeating: "My skin is healing a little more each day. My body knows how to return to balance."

"I felt silly at first," Robert admits. "But I committed to believing it could help. Within weeks, patches that had resisted every cream and medication for years began to clear. My dermatologist was stunned."

The Healing Power of Community

Another powerful mental factor in healing is social connection. Studies show that isolation increases inflammatory markers, while meaningful social bonds can reduce them.

Priya found this to be true after her lupus diagnosis left her feeling alienated from her former active life. While diligently following an anti-inflammatory nutrition plan, she joined a support group—not just to discuss symptoms, but to celebrate small victories and maintain positive focus.

"We made a pact to acknowledge struggles without letting them dominate our conversations," Priya explains. "We shared anti-inflammatory recipes, meditation techniques, and most importantly, we held space for each other's healing journeys."

This combination of nutritional changes and positive social connection led to such significant improvement that Priya's rheumatologist was able to reduce her medication dosage for the first time in years.

Building Your Healing Mindset

How can you harness the power of mind alongside nutrition for your own healing journey? Experts suggest several complementary approaches:

1. **Conscious Language:** Pay attention to how you speak about your condition, both aloud and in your thoughts. Replace "my disease" with "the inflammation I'm experiencing." This subtle shift acknowledges the condition without claiming it as an intrinsic part of your identity.
2. **Visualization:** Spend time daily imagining your body in a state of healing. Be specific — picture anti-inflammatory foods calming overactive immune responses or reducing oxidative stress.
3. **Stress Management:** Recognize that stress reduction isn't a luxury but a medical necessity for inflammatory conditions. Find practices that resonate with you, whether that's breathing exercises, gentle movement, or creative expression.
4. **Expectation Setting:** Cultivate genuine belief in your capacity for improvement. This doesn't mean denying current symptoms, but rather holding space for the possibility of feeling better.
5. **Gratitude Practice:** Acknowledge what your body can do rather than focusing exclusively on limitations. This shifts your nervous system from fight-or-flight to rest-and-repair.

A Holistic Approach

Sarah, whose story began this journey, ultimately found her path forward through this integrated approach. She began following the anti-inflammatory nutrition guidelines while simultaneously practicing mindfulness meditation and keeping a healing journal.

"I stopped seeing food as just food and my thoughts as just thoughts," Sarah reflects. "I began understanding them as information my body was processing — either inflammatory or anti-inflammatory information."

Six months into her practice, Sarah's inflammatory markers had decreased significantly. More importantly, her quality of life had transformed. "The pain isn't completely gone," she acknowledges, "but my relationship with it has changed fundamentally. I'm participating in my healing rather than just enduring my symptoms."

Dr. Martinez emphasizes that this mind-body approach doesn't replace conventional medical care but enhances it. "We need to move beyond the false dichotomy between physical and psychological approaches," she argues. "Your mind and body aren't separate entities—they're aspects of your whole being, constantly communicating and influencing each other."

As you explore the anti-inflammatory recipes in this cookbook, consider that you're not just changing what's on your plate, but potentially transforming your relationship with your body. Every nutritious meal becomes an act of self-compassion, a message to your cells that healing matters. Every mindful moment becomes an opportunity to shift from stress to restoration.

The most powerful medicine may be this integration—honoring the inseparable connection between what we eat and how we think, between caring for our bodies and calming our minds. In this holistic approach, we find not just the management of symptoms but the possibility of profound healing.

The Complete Guide Of Building Your Healing Mindset

When Clara first received her diagnosis of rheumatoid arthritis at age 36, she felt as though her life had been divided into "before" and "after." The pain and fatigue seemed to shrink her world, and despite following her doctor's recommendations meticulously, she continued to struggle.

"I was doing everything right with my medications and diet," Clara recalls. "But I still felt like my body was my enemy. Every morning, I'd wake up dreading how I would feel."

Clara's story is common among those facing inflammatory conditions. While nutrition and medical interventions form crucial foundations for healing, many discover that lasting improvement requires a third component: a deliberate reshaping of mental patterns and beliefs about health, pain, and recovery.

Understanding the Mind-Inflammation Connection

Dr. Nathan Rivera, psychoneuroimmunologist at Stanford University, explains: "The communication between brain and immune system is bidirectional. Inflammatory cytokines can trigger depressive symptoms and brain fog, while psychological stress can increase inflammation. Breaking this cycle often requires intervening at both levels simultaneously."

This understanding becomes the cornerstone of building a healing mindset. It's not about positive thinking as a magical cure, but rather about recognizing that your thoughts and emotions create real biochemical responses that can either support or hinder your healing journey.

Awareness: The First Step

Like Clara, Jerome had been diligently following an anti-inflammatory diet for his psoriatic arthritis with moderate success. His breakthrough began with a simple journaling exercise suggested by his integrative medicine doctor.

"She asked me to write down what went through my mind when I experienced a flare-up," Jerome explains. "I was shocked to discover how catastrophic my thinking became. One painful joint would lead to thoughts like, 'I'll never get better,' or 'This will only get worse.'"

This awareness allowed Jerome to recognize how these thought patterns triggered stress responses, potentially worsening inflammation. Simply noticing these thoughts — without judgment — became his first step toward a new relationship with his condition.

Practice: Thought Awareness Journal Set aside 10 minutes daily to record thoughts that arise around your health, particularly during symptom flares. Note patterns without trying to change them immediately. This mindful observation creates space between you and automatic negative thoughts.

Reframing: Changing the Narrative

After becoming aware of her thoughts, Clara began working with a health psychologist who introduced her to cognitive reframing — the practice of consciously shifting perspective on situations.

"I learned to catch myself when I'd think, 'I can't handle this pain,'" Clara shares. "Instead, I'd reframe it as, 'I'm experiencing discomfort right now, and I have tools to manage it.'"

This subtle shift moves from helplessness to agency, from permanence to temporariness. Research shows that such reframing can reduce stress hormone production, potentially lowering inflammatory markers.

Mei, who struggled with inflammatory bowel disease, developed her own powerful reframe: "Instead of thinking, 'My body is attacking itself,' which made me feel betrayed, I began thinking, 'My immune system is working too hard to protect me.' This helped me feel compassion rather than anger toward my body."

Practice: The Reframing Technique When you notice a distressing thought about your health:

1. Write down the thought exactly as it occurs
2. Identify the emotion it produces (fear, anger, hopelessness)
3. Question its accuracy: Is this absolutely true? Am I seeing the whole picture?
4. Create an alternative view that acknowledges difficulty while incorporating hope and agency
5. Notice how the new perspective feels in your body

Visualization: Directing Your Inner Imagery

The mind naturally creates images — but often, with chronic inflammation, these images center around pain, limitation, or deterioration. Conscious visualization redirects this powerful faculty toward healing.

Marcus, who lived with ankylosing spondylitis for decades, discovered visualization through an unexpected source — his young daughter.

"She asked why I looked so sad about my 'ouchy back,'" Marcus remembers. "I told her my immune system was confused and attacking my spine. She suggested I should 'tell it a bedtime story so it doesn't feel scared anymore.' Something about her childlike wisdom struck me."

Marcus developed a daily 10-minute practice imagining his immune system as a confused guardian that needed gentle guidance rather than an enemy to be battled. He visualized calm, coordinated immune cells working properly while sending feelings of appreciation to his body.

"Combined with my anti-inflammatory diet, this practice marked a turning point," Marcus says. "My inflammation markers began decreasing steadily for the first time in years."

Practice: Healing Visualization Find a quiet space and comfortable position. Close your eyes and breathe deeply. Imagine:

1. Your immune system as a complex, intelligent network that's working to find balance
2. Anti-inflammatory foods you consume transforming into golden light that soothes inflamed areas
3. Each breath bringing oxygen to areas that need healing
4. Tension and inflammation gradually releasing with each exhale
5. Your cells remembering their natural, healthy state

Practice for 5-15 minutes daily, especially before meals to enhance the mind-body connection with your anti-inflammatory nutrition.

Body Awareness and Acceptance

Diana had been avoiding physical movement since her fibromyalgia diagnosis, fearing it would trigger more pain. Working with a mindfulness-based physical therapist introduced her to a different approach: gentle, curious attention to bodily sensations.

"I'd been either ignoring my body entirely or hyperfocusing on pain," Diana explains. "I never just experienced sensations neutrally."

She began practicing body scans — systematically noticing sensations throughout her body without immediately labeling them as "good" or "bad." Gradually, this practice helped her distinguish between different types of sensations and respond appropriately rather than reactively.

"I discovered I could feel discomfort without automatically tensing against it, which often made it worse," she shares. "This created space for more movement, which ultimately decreased my overall pain levels."

Practice: The Compassionate Body Scan Lie comfortably with eyes closed. Slowly move your attention from feet to head, spending 20-30 seconds with each body region. For each area:

1. Notice sensations without labeling them (warmth, coolness, tingling, pressure)
2. If you find pain or discomfort, acknowledge it without resistance
3. Breathe into that area with an attitude of gentle curiosity
4. Offer that part of your body compassion, regardless of how it feels
5. Before moving attention to the next area, mentally thank that body part for its efforts

Setting Healing Intentions

Joseph, recovering from severe psoriasis, found that setting clear intentions transformed his approach to both diet and mindset practices.

"Every morning, I'd state my intention for health, not from a place of desperation but genuine expectation," Joseph explains. "Before meals, I'd pause to appreciate how these specific foods would support my healing."

This practice of conscious intention setting anchors your mind in possibility rather than limitation. It transforms anti-inflammatory eating from a restrictive diet to a deliberate act of self-care.

Practice: Daily Healing Intentions Each morning, place a hand over your heart and state: "Today, I set my intention toward healing and wholeness. I choose foods, thoughts, and actions that support my body's natural balance."

Before each meal, take three deep breaths and silently acknowledge: "I choose these foods as medicine for my body. They nourish my cells and reduce inflammation with each bite."

The Power of Self-Compassion

Perhaps the most transformative mindset shift comes through self-compassion—relating to yourself with the same kindness you would offer a loved one facing illness.

Elena struggled with lupus for years while maintaining a perfectionist approach to her health regimen. "I'd berate myself for any dietary slip, missed meditation, or symptom flare," she remembers. "I was essentially creating a stress response on top of my condition."

Working with a health coach, Elena learned that this harsh self-criticism actually triggered inflammatory responses that undermined her healing efforts. She began practicing deliberate self-compassion, especially during flares or setbacks.

Research by Dr. Kristin Neff at the University of Texas has shown that self-compassion reduces stress hormones and inflammatory markers more effectively than self-criticism or even neutral self-talk.

Practice: Self-Compassion During Difficult Moments
When experiencing a symptom flare, disappointment, or setback:

1. Place hands gently on your heart or another soothing location
2. Acknowledge suffering: "This is a moment of difficulty"
3. Recognize shared humanity: "Difficulty is part of living with this condition; I'm not alone"
4. Offer kindness: "May I be gentle with myself right now"
5. Ask: "What would I say to a dear friend experiencing this same situation?"

Creating Empowering Language Patterns

The words we use — both internally and externally — shape our experience of illness and healing. Angela, who faced mixed connective tissue disease, noticed how her language framed her relationship with her condition.

"I used to say 'my disease' or talk about 'fighting' my condition," Angela notes. "My counselor suggested I experiment with different language. Instead of 'my disease,' I started saying 'the inflammation I'm experiencing.' Instead of 'fighting,' I began using 'balancing' or 'healing.'"

These semantic shifts might seem minor, but they represent fundamental changes in how we conceptualize illness and recovery.

Practice: Language Transformation Review these common phrases and their empowering alternatives:

Instead of: "My disease is flaring up" Try: "I'm experiencing increased inflammation right now"

Instead of: "I can't do anything because of my pain" Try: "I'm choosing gentle activities that support my body today"

Instead of: "I'll always have this condition" Try: "My body is capable of remarkable healing and balance"

Instead of: "Why won't my pain go away?" Try: "What is my body trying to communicate right now?"

Notice how different phrasings feel in your body when you speak them aloud.

Celebrating Micro-Improvements

When battling chronic inflammation, progress often arrives in subtle ways that can go unnoticed if we're focused solely on complete symptom resolution.

Carlos, managing psoriatic arthritis, developed a practice of deliberately noting tiny improvements. "One day I realized I could turn the shower knob without wincing," he shares. "Another day, I noticed I wasn't thinking about pain during my morning meditation. These weren't dramatic changes, but acknowledging them built my confidence that healing was possible."

This practice of noticing and celebrating micro-improvements creates a positive feedback loop that supports continued healing.

Practice: The Progress Journal Keep a small notebook by your bed. Each evening, answer three questions:

1. What went well today regarding my health, however small?
2. What did my body accomplish today that I'm grateful for?
3. What subtle improvement have I noticed recently?

If you're having a particularly difficult day, adjust the third question to: "What hasn't gotten worse, even amid challenges?"

Navigating Setbacks With Resilience

Healing from inflammatory conditions rarely follows a linear path. Even with the most careful nutrition and mindset practices, setbacks can occur. The difference between those who continue improving and those who plateau often lies in how they respond to these inevitable fluctuations.

Leila, managing endometriosis, developed what she calls her "setback protocol" after working with a health psychologist.

"Previously, a symptom flare would send me into despair," Leila explains. "Now I have a mental framework ready. I acknowledge disappointment without spiraling, review possible triggers without blame, and reconnect with practices that have helped before."

Practice: The Resilience Response When experiencing a setback:

1. Acknowledge emotions without judgment: "I feel disappointed and concerned, and that's natural"
2. Remind yourself of the non-linear nature of healing: "Fluctuations are normal and don't erase progress"
3. Get curious rather than critical: "What might my body need right now?"

4. Return to foundational practices: nutrition, rest, gentle movement, stress management
5. Reach out for support rather than isolating
6. Remember previous improvements as evidence of your body's capacity to heal

Synergy Between Nutrition and Mindset

Dr. Sophia Chen, who specializes in integrative approaches to autoimmune conditions, emphasizes that nutrition and mindset work synergistically rather than separately.

"The most profound healing I've witnessed occurs when patients approach anti-inflammatory eating with mindfulness and intention," Dr. Chen explains. "The act of consciously choosing healing foods actually enhances their biochemical effects through reduced stress hormones and improved digestion."

Clara, whose story began this section, ultimately discovered this synergy. She began taking a moment before meals to express gratitude for the healing properties of her food. She visualized anti-inflammatory compounds reducing her joint inflammation. She practiced self-compassion when symptoms flared rather than blaming herself.

"Six months into this integrated approach, my rheumatologist was shocked by my improvement," Clara shares. "My inflammatory markers had dropped significantly, and more importantly, my quality of life had transformed. I still have rheumatoid arthritis, but my relationship with it—and with myself—has fundamentally changed."

Your Mindset Toolkit

As you embark on your anti-inflammatory nutrition journey, consider this mindset toolkit essential equipment for your path:

1. **Awareness** of thought patterns that increase stress and potentially inflammation
2. **Reframing** perspectives to support healing rather than hopelessness
3. **Visualization** of your body's innate healing capacity
4. **Body awareness** that allows you to respond to needs with compassion
5. **Intention setting** that directs your mind toward healing possibilities
6. **Self-compassion** that reduces stress responses during challenges
7. **Empowering language** that shapes your relationship with health and healing
8. **Celebrating micro-improvements** to build confidence in healing
9. **Resilience practices** for navigating inevitable fluctuations

Remember that building a healing mindset isn't about forcing positivity or denying difficulties. Rather, it's about cultivating a relationship with your body based on partnership rather than battle, possibility rather than limitation, and compassion rather than criticism.

Combined with the nourishing anti-inflammatory recipes in this book, these mindset practices offer a comprehensive approach to managing inflammation and reclaiming vibrant health — one thought, one bite, one day at a time.

Creating Your Personalized Mind-Body Healing Protocol

After six months of combining anti-inflammatory nutrition with mindfulness practices, Thomas noticed something surprising: certain foods affected him differently depending on his mental state.

"When I ate under stress, even the healthiest anti-inflammatory meals would sometimes trigger symptoms," Thomas explains. "But when I ate the same foods in a calm, present state, my body seemed to process them differently."

This observation highlights a crucial aspect of healing: the mind-body connection isn't just a concept—it's a practical reality that influences how we respond to everything from nutrition to medication.

The Stress-Digestion Connection

Dr. Amira Hashmi, gastroenterologist and researcher on the gut-brain axis, explains: "Stress activates the sympathetic nervous system—our 'fight or flight' response—which diverts blood away from digestive organs. This can impair nutrient absorption, alter gut permeability, and change how we metabolize even the healthiest foods."

This understanding opens a new dimension to anti-inflammatory healing: learning to activate the parasympathetic "rest and digest" state before meals maximizes the benefits of your carefully chosen nutrition.

Practice: The Pre-Meal Reset Before each meal:

1. Take 3-5 deep belly breaths, extending your exhales longer than your inhales

2. Place one hand on your abdomen and silently say, "I am now entering digestive mode"
3. Take a moment to visually appreciate the colors and nourishment on your plate
4. Express gratitude for how these foods will support your healing
5. Take your first bite with full attention, noticing flavors and textures

Many practitioners report this simple 60-second practice significantly reduces post-meal discomfort and enhances the anti-inflammatory benefits of their nutrition.

Advanced Emotional Processing for Inflammation Reduction

While basic mindfulness helps manage emotional responses, many people with inflammatory conditions benefit from deeper emotional processing work. Research increasingly suggests that unresolved emotional experiences may maintain chronic stress responses that contribute to inflammation.

Lucia had followed an anti-inflammatory diet meticulously for her psoriasis but reached a plateau in her improvement. Working with a somatic experiencing practitioner, she began addressing childhood experiences that had created persistent patterns of threat response in her nervous system.

"I discovered that my body was still carrying old stress patterns that kept triggering inflammatory cascades," Lucia shares. "Learning to recognize and release these patterns through body-centered emotional processing created another level of healing."

Practice: Emotional Body Mapping This practice helps identify where emotions may be stored as physical tension:

1. Sit or lie comfortably with eyes closed

2. Scan your body systematically from head to toe
3. Notice areas of tension, discomfort, or numbness
4. For each area, gently ask: "What emotion might be held here?"
5. Without judgment, allow any images, memories, or sensations to arise
6. Place a hand on that area and breathe into it with compassion
7. Silently say: "I acknowledge what's held here and allow it to release"

For deeper emotional processing, consider working with a qualified therapist specializing in somatic approaches like Somatic Experiencing, EMDR, or Sensorimotor Psychotherapy.

The Healing Power of Nature Connection

Environmental factors play a significant role in inflammation, but research shows that positive nature exposure can reduce inflammatory markers and stress hormones while enhancing immune function.

After years of managing Crohn's disease, Sophia noticed her symptoms improved dramatically during a forest vacation. Intrigued, she began incorporating regular "forest bathing" (the Japanese practice of shinrin-yoku) into her health routine.

"Fifteen minutes among trees seemed to calm my gut in ways that even my medications couldn't always achieve," Sophia explains. "Now it's a non-negotiable part of my anti-inflammatory lifestyle alongside nutrition."

Studies from Japan and Scandinavia confirm that forest environments can reduce cortisol levels by up to 40% and decrease inflammatory cytokines — potentially through plant compounds called phytoncides and the sensory richness of natural settings.

Practice: Healing Nature Immersion Even if you have limited mobility or access to nature:

1. Find any natural setting — a park, garden, or even a window view of trees
2. Engage all five senses deliberately: notice colors, textures, sounds, scents
3. Touch natural elements if possible — bark, leaves, grass, stones
4. Breathe deeply, imagining plant-produced compounds entering your lungs
5. Mentally connect with the resilience of natural systems — growth, regeneration, adaptation
6. Spend at least 15 minutes in this sensory immersion

For those with severe mobility limitations, research shows that even viewing nature photographs or listening to nature sounds produces measurable anti-inflammatory effects.

Sleep Optimization: The Ultimate Anti-Inflammatory

While nutrition receives significant attention in inflammatory conditions, sleep quality may be equally crucial. During deep sleep, the body performs essential anti-inflammatory processes and tissue repair that cannot occur during wakefulness.

Jason struggled with psoriatic arthritis for years while also battling insomnia. "I was doing everything right with diet but sleeping only 4-5 hours a night," he recalls. "When I finally addressed my sleep, my inflammatory markers dropped more in two months than they had in two years of dietary changes alone."

Practice: The Anti-Inflammatory Sleep Protocol Beyond basic sleep hygiene, these practices specifically support inflammatory healing:

1. **Temperature regulation**: Keep your bedroom cool (65-68°F/18-20°C) — studies show this reduces nighttime inflammation
2. **Consistent timing**: Go to bed and wake at the same times to optimize cortisol rhythms
3. **Darkness immersion**: Use blackout curtains and eliminate all light sources — even dim light disrupts melatonin, which has anti-inflammatory properties
4. **Pre-sleep unwinding**: Create a 30-minute buffer between screens/stimulation and sleep
5. **Sleep position awareness**: If you have localized inflammation, experiment with positions that reduce pressure on affected areas
6. **Evening anti-inflammatory support**: Consider inflammation-calming teas like turmeric, ginger, or chamomile as part of your bedtime routine

For persistent sleep difficulties, consider consulting a sleep specialist — improving this fundamental aspect of health can dramatically enhance your body's response to anti-inflammatory nutrition.

Movement as Medicine: Finding Your Balance

Physical activity presents a paradox for many with inflammatory conditions: too little increases systemic inflammation, while too much can trigger flares. The key lies in finding personalized movement that calms rather than exacerbates inflammation.

After years of attempting high-intensity exercise that left her fibromyalgia worse, Eliza discovered that gentle, mindful movement produced better results. "I switched from pushing through pain to moving with awareness," she explains. "Walking in nature, tai chi, and specific yoga sequences actually reduced my pain instead of increasing it."

Practice: Inflammation-Responsive Movement This approach honors your body's changing needs:

1. Before moving, take 30 seconds to scan your body and assess inflammation levels
2. Set an intention: "I move to support healing, not to push through pain"
3. Begin with 5 minutes of gentle movement, then reassess how your body feels
4. If symptoms decrease, continue; if they increase, modify or rest
5. Focus on quality of movement rather than quantity or intensity
6. Include range-of-motion exercises for affected joints
7. End with 2-3 minutes of conscious relaxation

Remember that appropriate movement increases circulation of anti-inflammatory compounds from your nutrition while reducing stress hormones—making it a powerful complement to dietary approaches.

Community and Connection: The Social Dimension of Healing

While personal mindset work is powerful, research increasingly shows that social connections significantly influence inflammatory levels. Studies find that social isolation increases inflammatory markers comparable to smoking or obesity, while meaningful connection reduces them.

Mark had followed a strict anti-inflammatory protocol for ankylosing spondylitis but struggled with feelings of isolation. Joining a support group — not just for information but for genuine connection — marked a turning point.

"Something changed when I stopped facing this alone," Mark shares. "Our group meals featuring anti-inflammatory recipes became powerful healing experiences beyond just the nutrition."

Practice: Healing Connection Cultivation To harness the anti-inflammatory power of connection:

1. Identify at least one person with whom you can share your health journey authentically
2. Consider joining a support group (in-person or online) specific to your condition
3. Practice vulnerability — appropriate sharing of challenges builds meaningful connection
4. Balance health discussions with other topics to maintain multidimensional relationships
5. Share anti-inflammatory meals with others when possible — research shows eating in community enhances digestion and nutrient absorption
6. Offer support to others, which research shows activates reward centers in the brain that reduce inflammation

Creating Your Personalized Protocol

After exploring various mindset approaches, many people wonder which to prioritize. The answer lies in personalization — discovering which practices most effectively complement your anti-inflammatory nutrition.

Aiden, managing ulcerative colitis, created a system to identify his most effective practices. "I developed a simple tracking method," he explains. "After each practice, I'd rate my symptoms and energy levels. Within weeks, clear patterns emerged showing which approaches helped most."

Practice: The Personal Effectiveness Tracker For two weeks:

1. List all mindset and lifestyle practices you're considering
2. After each practice, rate symptom levels before and after (1-10 scale)
3. Note energy levels and overall wellbeing (1-10 scale)
4. Record any observations about sleep quality, digestion, or mood
5. After two weeks, review your data to identify your "power practices" — those that consistently show positive effects
6. Create a sustainable routine prioritizing these evidence-based personal practices

Dr. Rivera emphasizes that this personalization is crucial: "What works for one person's inflammatory profile may differ from another's. By tracking responses, you become a scientist of your own healing journey."

Navigating Healthcare with a Mindset of Partnership

Many people with inflammatory conditions struggle with medical interactions, often feeling unheard or dismissed. Developing a partnership mindset can transform these experiences from stressful to supportive.

After years of difficult doctor appointments, Elena shifted her approach. "I stopped seeing doctors as authorities who should 'fix' me and started viewing them as specialized consultants on my healing team," she explains. "This changed everything about those interactions."

Practice: The Partnership Preparation Before medical appointments:

1. Document specific symptoms, timing, and potential triggers
2. Prioritize 2-3 key questions or concerns
3. Prepare a brief summary of what you've tried and results observed
4. Set an intention: "I am an active participant in this exchange"
5. Practice articulating your experiences clearly and concisely
6. Bring someone to support you if appointments typically feel overwhelming

This approach reduces the stress of medical interactions — important since appointment-related stress can actually trigger inflammatory flares in sensitive individuals.

Integrating Spirituality and Meaning

For many, healing from chronic inflammation involves not just physical and mental dimensions but spiritual ones as well. Research shows that a sense of meaning and purpose correlates with lower inflammatory markers, regardless of specific religious beliefs.

Daniel, managing rheumatoid arthritis, found that connecting his health journey to deeper values transformed his experience. "When I reframed my condition as an opportunity to develop compassion and help others, something shifted," he shares. "The suffering became meaningful rather than just senseless, and paradoxically, my symptoms began improving."

Practice: Finding Meaning in the Journey To explore the spiritual dimension of healing:

1. Reflect on how your health journey has changed your perspective on life
2. Identify values that have become more important through this experience
3. Consider ways your insights might benefit others facing similar challenges
4. Connect with traditions or practices that provide spiritual nourishment
5. Explore how your health practices (nutrition, mindfulness) might align with deeper values and beliefs
6. Journal on the question: "How might this experience be serving my growth or understanding?"

Many find that this meaning-making process reduces the stress of uncertainty and provides emotional resilience during difficult phases of healing.

The Continuous Journey

As you integrate these advanced mindset practices with your anti-inflammatory nutrition, remember that healing is not a destination but a continuous journey of discovery and adaptation.

Mira, who has managed lupus for fifteen years, shares: "I used to think healing meant becoming the person I was before my diagnosis. Now I understand it's about becoming someone new — more aware, more compassionate, more intentional about how I live. My relationship with food, with my body, with stress — it's all transformed."

This perspective reflects the ultimate mindset shift: from seeing inflammatory conditions as obstacles to overcome to recognizing them as catalysts for profound transformation. The symptoms that once seemed like your greatest burden may ultimately guide you toward your greatest wisdom.

Dr. Hashmi offers this perspective: "In integrative medicine, we see that those who heal most profoundly are often those who use their condition as an invitation to live differently — not just eating anti-inflammatory foods but cultivating anti-inflammatory thoughts, relationships, and life choices."

As you continue exploring the recipes and recommendations in this book, carry this understanding with you: each meal becomes more powerful when prepared with intention, each mindset practice more effective when connected to nourishing nutrition, each day an opportunity to align body, mind, and spirit in the direction of healing.

The path may not always be linear, but with this integrated approach, it will invariably lead toward greater balance, resilience, and wellbeing — one thought, one breath, one nourishing bite at a time.

Importance of Gut Health in Autoimmunity

1. The gut plays a crucial role in immune system function and overall health. In fact, an increasing body of research suggests that gut health is intricately linked to the development and progression of autoimmune diseases. Understanding this connection is essential for addressing the underlying factors contributing to autoimmunity.
2. The Gut-Immune System Connection

3. The gut is home to a complex ecosystem of trillions of microorganisms, collectively known as the gut microbiome. This diverse community of bacteria, viruses, and fungi plays a vital role in digestion, nutrient absorption, and immune system regulation.
4. The gut is also a crucial component of the body's immune system, housing a significant portion of immune cells. The gut-associated lymphoid tissue (GALT) is responsible for recognizing and responding to potential threats, such as pathogens or harmful substances, while also maintaining tolerance to harmless substances like food particles.
5. When the delicate balance of the gut microbiome is disrupted, a condition known as dysbiosis can occur. Dysbiosis is linked to increased intestinal permeability (leaky gut), allowing partially digested food particles, toxins, and bacteria to enter the bloodstream. This can trigger an immune response, leading to inflammation and potentially contributing to the development of autoimmune diseases.
6. Factors that can contribute to gut dysbiosis and autoimmunity include:
7.
8. Diet: Consuming a diet high in processed foods, refined carbohydrates, and unhealthy fats can disrupt the gut microbiome and promote inflammation.
9. Antibiotics and medications: While necessary in some cases, the overuse of antibiotics can deplete beneficial gut bacteria, paving the way for dysbiosis.
10. Stress: Chronic stress can alter gut motility, increase intestinal permeability, and disrupt the balance of gut microbes.
11. Environmental toxins: Exposure to pesticides, heavy metals, and other environmental toxins can contribute to gut inflammation and dysbiosis.
12. Infections: Certain viral, bacterial, or parasitic infections can disrupt gut health and potentially trigger an autoimmune response.

13.
14. The Autoimmune Protocol (AIP) Diet and Gut Health
15. The AIP diet is designed to address gut health by removing potentially inflammatory and gut-disrupting foods while promoting the consumption of nutrient-dense, gut-healing foods. By eliminating grains, legumes, dairy, and other potential triggers, the AIP diet aims to reduce intestinal inflammation and promote a balanced gut microbiome.
16. Additionally, the AIP diet emphasizes the consumption of fermented foods, bone broth, and other gut-nourishing foods that can support the growth of beneficial gut bacteria and aid in the healing of the gut lining.
17. While more research is needed to fully understand the complex relationship between gut health and autoimmunity, the AIP diet's focus on promoting a healthy gut environment may play a crucial role in managing autoimmune conditions and supporting overall immune system function.

Basics of Autoimmune Protocol (AIP) Diet

The Autoimmune Protocol (AIP) diet is an elimination diet designed to help manage autoimmune conditions by reducing inflammation and promoting gut health. It involves removing certain food groups that are commonly associated with triggering immune system reactions and promoting the consumption of nutrient-dense, anti-inflammatory foods.

The Elimination Phase

The first phase of the AIP diet involves eliminating the following food groups:

Grains (including gluten-containing grains like wheat, barley, and rye)
Legumes (beans, lentils, peanuts, and peanut products)
Dairy products
Eggs
Nightshade vegetables (tomatoes, potatoes, eggplants, peppers)
Nuts and seeds
Refined sugars and processed foods
Non-nutritive sweeteners (e.g., artificial sweeteners)
Alcohol

Advantage and Potential Risks of Aip

These foods are eliminated because they are known to be common triggers for inflammation, gut irritation, and immune system reactions in individuals with autoimmune conditions.
The AIP-Friendly Foods
While the AIP diet may seem restrictive, there is still a wide variety of nutrient-dense, anti-inflammatory foods that are encouraged:

Vegetables (excluding nightshades)
Fruits
Quality proteins (grass-fed meats, wild-caught fish, and seafood)
Healthy fats (olive oil, avocado oil, coconut oil, animal fats)
Bone broth

Fermented foods (sauerkraut, kimchi, coconut yogurt)
Herbs and spices (excluding seed-based spices)
Green tea and herbal teas

These foods are rich in essential nutrients, antioxidants, and anti-inflammatory compounds that support gut health, immune system function, and overall well-being.

The Reintroduction Phase

After following the elimination phase for a period of time (typically 30-90 days), the reintroduction phase begins. During this phase, eliminated foods are slowly reintroduced one at a time, allowing for the identification of potential food triggers. This process is crucial for determining which foods may need to be avoided long-term and which can be reintroduced without adverse reactions.

It's important to note that the AIP diet is not a one-size-fits-all approach, and individual responses may vary. Working with a qualified healthcare professional, such as a nutritionist or functional medicine practitioner, can help guide the implementation and personalization of the AIP diet for optimal results.

Getting Started

- Making the transition to the Autoimmune Protocol (AIP) Diet can seem daunting at first, but with proper planning and preparation, it can become a manageable and sustainable lifestyle change. This chapter will provide practical tips and strategies for successfully implementing the AIP diet.

Clear Off Your Pantry and Fridge

The first step in starting the AIP diet is to remove all non-compliant foods from your kitchen. This includes:

Grains (wheat, barley, rye, oats, corn, etc.)
Legumes (beans, lentils, peanuts, soy)
Dairy products
Eggs
Nightshade vegetables (tomatoes, potatoes, eggplants, peppers)
Nuts and seeds
Refined sugars and processed foods
Non-nutritive sweeteners
Alcohol

Carefully read ingredient labels and discard or donate any items that contain these ingredients. This step is crucial to eliminate temptation and ensure a clean slate for your AIP journey.

Stocking Up on AIP-Friendly Foods

Once you've cleared out your pantry and fridge, it's time to restock with AIP-compliant foods. Here are some essential items to have on hand:

Vegetables (leafy greens, cruciferous veggies, carrots, beets, etc.)
Fruits (berries, citrus, avocados, bananas, etc.)
Quality proteins (grass-fed meats, wild-caught fish, and seafood)
Healthy fats (olive oil, avocado oil, coconut oil, ghee)
Bone broth
Fermented foods (sauerkraut, kimchi, coconut yogurt)
Herbs and spices (excluding seed-based spices)
Green tea and herbal teas
AIP-friendly condiments (coconut aminos, fruit-based vinegars, etc.)

Meal Planning and Preparation

Proper meal planning and preparation are key to successfully following the AIP diet. Consider the following tips:

Create a weekly meal plan: Plan out your meals and snacks for the week, taking into account any social events or activities that may require additional preparation.

Batch cooking: Set aside time to batch cook AIP-friendly meals and snacks for the week, which can save time and ensure you have compliant options readily available.

Involve the family: If you're cooking for a family, involve them in the process and adapt family-favorite recipes to be AIP-compliant. This can help ensure everyone's needs are met and increase compliance.

Prepare for dining out: Research restaurants in your area that offer AIP-friendly options or call ahead to inquire about accommodations. Pack AIP-compliant snacks or meals when necessary.

Stay organized: Keep a well-stocked pantry and fridge, and consider using meal prep containers or freezer-safe bags to store pre-portioned meals and snacks.

Adapting Family Favorites to AIP

One of the challenges of following the AIP diet is finding ways to adapt beloved family recipes to fit the dietary guidelines. Here are some tips for modifying traditional recipes:

Swap out non-compliant ingredients: Replace grains with AIP-friendly alternatives like cauliflower rice, zucchini noodles, or sweet potato noodles. Use coconut milk or nut-free milk alternatives instead of dairy.

Explore new cooking techniques: Experiment with cooking methods like baking, roasting, or grilling to create delicious AIP-compliant dishes.

Get creative with seasonings: Use a variety of AIP-friendly herbs, spices, and condiments to add flavor and depth to your dishes.

Be patient and keep an open mind: It may take some trial and error to find AIP-friendly recipes that satisfy your taste preferences. Stay open to trying new ingredients and flavor combinations.

By following these tips and strategies, you can successfully transition to the Autoimmune Protocol (AIP) Diet and set yourself up for long-term success in managing your autoimmune condition through dietary interventions.

A List of AIP-Friendly Foods

Following the Autoimmune Protocol (AIP) diet can be challenging, especially when you're first starting out. To help make the transition smoother, it's essential to familiarize yourself with the wide variety of foods that are permitted on the AIP diet. This chapter provides a comprehensive list of AIP-friendly foods to help you plan your meals and ensure you're getting a well-rounded, nutrient-dense diet.
Vegetables (excluding nightshades)

Leafy greens (spinach, kale, arugula, Swiss chard)
Cruciferous veggies (broccoli, cauliflower, Brussels sprouts, cabbage)
Root veggies (carrots, beets, parsnips, turnips)
Squash (zucchini, yellow squash, butternut squash, acorn squash)
Onions, garlic, leeks, shallots
Mushrooms
Asparagus, artichokes, okra

Cucumbers, celery, radishes

Fruits

Berries (strawberries, blueberries, raspberries, blackberries)
Citrus fruits (oranges, lemons, limes, grapefruit)
Apples, pears, peaches, plums
Bananas, plantains
Avocados
Melon (watermelon, cantaloupe, honeydew)
Mango, pineapple

Quality Proteins

Grass-fed beef, bison, lamb
Wild-caught fish and seafood (salmon, cod, shrimp, tuna)
Pasture-raised poultry (chicken, turkey)
Organ meats (liver, heart, tongue)
Wild game (venison, elk, boar)

Healthy Fats

Avocado oil, olive oil, coconut oil
Ghee (clarified butter)
Animal fats (tallow, lard from AIP sources)
Coconut butter/manna
Olives

Herbs and Spices

Fresh herbs (basil, cilantro, parsley, rosemary, thyme)
Dried herbs and spices (excluding seed-based spices like cumin, coriander)
Ginger, turmeric, garlic powder, onion powder

Beverages

Water
Herbal teas (chamomile, ginger, peppermint)
Green tea
Bone broth
Coconut milk (unsweetened)
Fruit-infused waters

Fermented Foods

Sauerkraut
Kimchi
Coconut yogurt
Kombucha (without added sweeteners)

Condiments and Seasonings

Apple cider vinegar
Coconut aminos
Fruit-based vinegars (balsamic, red wine)
Mustard powder
Fresh herbs and spices
Sea salt, black pepper

By familiarizing yourself with this comprehensive list of AIP-friendly foods, you'll be better equipped to create delicious and nutrient-dense meals that support your autoimmune health journey. Remember, it's also essential to work closely with a qualified healthcare professional to ensure that the AIP diet is tailored to your specific needs and health goals.

Chapter 1: Breakfast and Brunch AIP Diet Recipes

Sweet Potato Hash

Prep Time: 15 minutes
Cook Time: 25 minutes
Total Time: 40 minutes
Servings: 4
Ingredients:

2 medium sweet potatoes, diced into 1/2-inch cubes (about 4 cups)
1 red bell pepper, diced
1 yellow onion, diced
4 oz mushrooms, sliced
2 cloves garlic, minced
2 tbsp avocado oil or olive oil
1 tsp paprika
1/2 tsp sea salt
1/4 tsp black pepper
4 cups baby spinach or arugula
Optional protein: 4 cooked AIP breakfast sausage patties or 8 oz chicken, diced

Instructions:

Preheat oven to 400°F. Toss the diced sweet potatoes with 1 tbsp of the oil and spread out on a baking sheet. Roast for 20 minutes until fork tender.
In a large skillet, heat the remaining 1 tbsp oil over medium-high heat. Add the bell pepper, onion, mushrooms and garlic. Saute for 5-7 minutes until softened.
Add the roasted sweet potatoes, paprika, salt, pepper and spinach/arugula. Toss everything together until the greens are wilted.
If adding protein, fold in the cooked sausage or chicken now.

Serve the sweet potato hash warm.

Nutrition per serving (1/4th of recipe without added protein):
Calories: 204
Carbs: 28g
Fiber: 5g
Protein: 3g
Fat: 9g
This sweet potato hash is packed with vitamin A, vitamin C, iron and antioxidants from the veggies. Adding a protein makes it a complete, satisfying meal. It's AIP-compliant, nutrient-dense and delicious! Let me know if you need anything else on this recipe.

Coconut Flour Pancakes

Prep Time: 10 minutes
Cook Time: 15 minutes
Total Time: 25 minutes
Servings: 4 (makes 8 pancakes)
Ingredients:

1/2 cup coconut flour
1/2 tsp baking soda
1/4 tsp sea salt
4 eggs
1/2 cup coconut milk (from a carton, not canned)
2 tbsp maple syrup
1 tsp apple cider vinegar
1 tsp vanilla extract
2 tbsp coconut oil or avocado oil, plus more for cooking

Instructions:

In a medium bowl, whisk together the coconut flour, baking soda and salt.

In a separate bowl, whisk together the eggs, coconut milk, maple syrup, vinegar and vanilla.

Pour the wet ingredients into the dry and whisk until fully combined and no lumps remain. Let batter rest for 5 minutes to thicken.

Heat a non-stick skillet or griddle over medium heat and grease with coconut/avocado oil.

Pour 1/4 cup portions of the batter onto the hot surface and cook for 2-3 minutes until bubbles form on the surface.

Flip and cook another 1-2 minutes until golden brown on both sides. Repeat with remaining batter.

Serve the coconut flour pancakes warm with desired AIP-friendly toppings like maple syrup, fruit, cinnamon or coconut butter.

Nutrition per serving (2 pancakes without toppings):
Calories: 261
Total Carbs: 17g
Fiber: 8g
Protein: 7g
Fat: 19g
These grain-free coconut flour pancakes are fluffier and higher in fiber than regular pancakes. They are satisfying yet nutrient-dense, making them an AIP-friendly breakfast treat.

Zucchini Noodles with Pesto

Prep Time: 20 minutes
Cook Time: 5 minutes
Total Time: 25 minutes
Servings: 4
Ingredients:
For the Zucchini Noodles:

4 medium zucchinis, spiralized into noodles
1 tbsp avocado oil or olive oil

For the Pesto:

2 cups fresh basil leaves
1/2 cup olive oil
1/4 cup nutritional yeast
2 cloves garlic
1/4 cup pine nuts
2 tbsp lemon juice
1/2 tsp sea salt
1/4 tsp black pepper

Instructions:

Make the pesto by adding the basil, olive oil, nutritional yeast, garlic, pine nuts, lemon juice, salt and pepper to a food processor or blender. Pulse until well combined but still slightly chunky. Scrape down sides as needed.
Heat the 1 tbsp oil in a large skillet over medium-high heat. Add the zucchini noodles and sauté for 2-3 minutes until just tender but still crisp.

Remove zucchini noodles from heat and toss with the fresh pesto until fully coated.
Serve the zucchini noodle pesto immediately, garnished with extra pine nuts and basil if desired.

Nutrition per serving (1/4th of recipe):
Calories: 325
Total Carbs: 14g
Fiber: 4g
Protein: 7g
Fat: 29g
This light and fresh zucchini noodle dish is packed with healthy fats, fiber, vitamins and minerals. The zucchini noodles make it low-carb while the vibrant basil pesto adds tons of flavor. It's an easy, delicious AIP meal.

Chicken and Vegetable Stir-Fry

Prep Time: 15 minutes
Cook Time: 15 minutes
Total Time: 30 minutes
Servings: 4
Ingredients:

2 tbsp avocado oil or coconut oil
1 yellow onion, sliced
8 oz mushrooms, sliced
2 cups shredded cabbage or cole slaw mix
2 cups baby spinach
2 cloves garlic, minced
1 lb chicken breast or thighs, diced into 1-inch pieces
2 tsp coconut aminos
1 tsp toasted sesame oil
Sea salt and pepper to taste

Instructions:

Heat 1 tbsp of the avocado/coconut oil in a large skillet or wok over medium-high heat.
Add the diced chicken and sauté for 5-6 minutes until cooked through. Remove chicken from the pan and set aside.
Heat the remaining 1 tbsp oil in the same pan. Add the onions and mushrooms and stir-fry for 3-4 minutes.
Add the cabbage, spinach, and garlic. Continue stir-frying for 2-3 more minutes until cabbage is wilted.
Return the cooked chicken to the pan along with the coconut aminos and toasted sesame oil. Toss everything together.
Season with salt and pepper to taste.
Serve the veggie stir-fry warm.

Nutrition per serving (1/4th of recipe):

Calories: 284
Total Carbs: 11g
Fiber: 4g
Protein: 28g
Fat: 16g
This veggie-packed stir-fry is a nutritious way to start the day. It's loaded with antioxidants, fiber, and protein to keep you feeling energized. Feel free to swap the protein for turkey, beef, or leave it out for a veggie stir-fry.

Berry Smoothie Bowl

Here are the details for the Berry Smoothie Bowl recipe:
Berry Smoothie Bowl
Prep Time: 10 minutes
Total Time: 10 minutes
Servings: 2
Ingredients:

1 cup frozen mixed berries
1 frozen banana
1 cup coconut milk (from a carton)
1 tbsp coconut butter or coconut manna (optional)
1 tsp vanilla extract
1 scoop collagen peptides (optional)

Toppings:

Fresh berries
Shredded coconut
Sliced bananas
AIP-friendly granola
Hemp seeds

Instructions:

Add the frozen berries, frozen banana, coconut milk, coconut butter (if using), vanilla, and collagen peptides (if using) to a blender.
Blend on high speed until completely smooth and creamy, stopping to scrape down sides as needed.
Pour the smoothie into two bowls.
Top with desired toppings like fresh berries, shredded coconut, banana slices, AIP granola, and hemp seeds.
Serve smoothie bowls immediately.

Nutrition per serving (without toppings):
Calories: 175
Carbs: 21g
Fiber: 4g
Protein: 5g (10g with collagen)
Fat: 8g
Notes:

For a thicker consistency, use frozen cauliflower rice instead of banana.
Swap cashew or almond milk for coconut if not following AIP diet.
Add spinach or other greens for extra nutrients.

This berry smoothie bowl is bursting with antioxidants, fiber, and healthy fats to fuel your morning. It's creamy, delicious and easy to customize with your favorite AIP-friendly toppings. Enjoy it for a nutritious start to your day!

Turmeric Scrambled Eggs

Here are the details for the Turmeric Scrambled Eggs recipe:
Turmeric Scrambled Eggs
Prep Time: 10 minutes
Cook Time: 10 minutes
Total Time: 20 minutes
Servings: 2
Ingredients:

6 eggs
2 tbsp coconut milk or almond milk
1 tsp turmeric powder
1/2 tsp garlic powder
1/4 tsp sea salt
1/4 tsp black pepper
2 tsp avocado oil or olive oil
1/2 cup diced onion
1 cup baby spinach
2 slices AIP-compliant bacon or sausage patties, cooked and crumbled (optional)

Instructions:

In a small bowl, whisk together the eggs, coconut/almond milk, turmeric, garlic powder, salt, and pepper until fully combined.
Heat the oil in a non-stick skillet over medium heat. Add the diced onion and sauté for 2-3 minutes until translucent.
Add the baby spinach and continue cooking for 1 minute until wilted.
Pour in the egg mixture and use a spatula to gently scramble the eggs. Cook for 3-4 minutes, stirring frequently, until eggs are scrambled to your desired doneness.

Remove from heat and fold in the crumbled bacon or sausage, if using.
Serve the turmeric scrambled eggs immediately, garnished with extra black pepper or green onions if desired.

Nutrition per serving (1/2 of recipe without bacon/sausage):
Calories: 264
Total Carbs: 6g
Fiber: 1g
Protein: 16g
Fat: 20g
Notes:

Swap egg whites for whole eggs to reduce calories/fat.
Add diced tomatoes or bell peppers for extra veggies.
Top with avocado slices for added healthy fats.

These turmeric scrambled eggs are a nutrient powerhouse! The anti-inflammatory turmeric gives them a vibrant golden color and delicious flavor. Packed with protein, greens, and customizable with your favorite AIP meats or veggies.

AIP Breakfast Skillet

Prep Time: 15 minutes
Cook Time: 25 minutes
Total Time: 40 minutes
Servings: 4
Ingredients:

1 pound Yukon gold potatoes, diced into 1/2-inch cubes
1 tablespoon avocado oil or olive oil, plus more for potatoes
1/2 pound chicken breakfast sausage, casing removed if linked
1/2 yellow onion, diced
1 bell pepper, diced
8 ounces mushrooms, sliced
2 cups baby spinach or kale, chopped
8 eggs
Sea salt and black pepper to taste

Instructions:

Preheat oven to 400°F. Toss the diced potatoes with enough oil to coat and spread on a baking sheet. Roast for 20-25 minutes until fork tender.

In a large oven-safe skillet, heat the 1 tablespoon oil over medium heat. Add the sausage and cook for 5-6 minutes, breaking it up as it cooks, until browned and cooked through. Remove sausage to a plate.

In the same skillet, add the onion, bell pepper and mushrooms. Sauté for 5 minutes until softened.

Add the roasted potatoes, cooked sausage and spinach/kale. Stir to combine and create a well in the center of the skillet.

Crack the 8 eggs into the well. Transfer the skillet to the oven and bake for 10-12 minutes until the egg whites are set but the yolks are still runny.

Remove from oven, season with salt and pepper, and serve the skillet warm, scooping portions onto plates.

Nutrition per serving (1/4 of recipe):
Calories: 391
Carbs: 27g
Fiber: 4g
Protein: 22g
Fat: 23g

This loaded breakfast skillet is a delicious, all-in-one meal with protein, veggies, and egg yolks for healthy fats. It's hearty, nutritious and fully AIP-compliant. Feel free to customize with your preferred protein or veggies.

Smoked Salmon and Avocado Wrap

Prep Time: 15 minutes
Total Time: 15 minutes
Servings: 4
Ingredients:

2 large avocados
8 oz smoked wild-caught salmon, flaked or diced
1/4 cup finely diced red onion
2 tbsp fresh lemon juice
2 tbsp chopped fresh dill (or 1 tsp dried)
1 tbsp avocado oil or olive oil
1/4 tsp sea salt
1/8 tsp black pepper

Instructions:

Cut the avocados in half lengthwise and remove the pits. Use a spoon to scoop out a bit of the flesh to create a larger well.
In a medium bowl, gently toss together the smoked salmon, red onion, lemon juice, dill, oil, salt, and pepper.
Divide the smoked salmon mixture evenly among the 4 avocado halves, spooning it into the wells.
Optionally, you can serve the stuffed avocados with extra lemon wedges, dill, and/or AIP-friendly hot sauce like Bravado Ghost Pepper & Blueberry.

Nutrition per serving (1 stuffed avocado half):
Calories: 236
Total Carbs: 9g
Fiber: 5g
Protein: 13g

Fat: 19g

These smoked salmon stuffed avocado boats make a protein-packed and flavorful breakfast or brunch. They are quick, require no cooking, and are full of healthy fats and nutrients. Easily double or triple the recipe for meal prep.

Plantain Waffles

Prep Time: 10 minutes
Cook Time: 20 minutes
Total Time: 30 minutes
Servings: 4 (makes 8 waffles)
Ingredients:

2 green plantains, peeled and diced (about 2 cups)
4 eggs
1/4 cup coconut oil, melted, plus more for waffle iron
1 tsp vanilla extract
1/2 tsp baking soda
1/4 tsp sea salt
1/4 cup warm water (if needed to thin batter)

Instructions:

Preheat your waffle iron and grease it well with coconut oil.
In a blender or food processor, blend the diced plantains until a smooth puree forms.
Add in the eggs, melted coconut oil, vanilla, baking soda, and salt. Blend again until fully combined. If batter seems too thick, add in the warm water a bit at a time to thin it out.
Pour batter onto the heated waffle iron in batches, using about 1/2 cup per waffle section. Close and cook for 5-7 minutes until golden brown and cooked through.
Remove waffles carefully and place on a wire rack or baking sheet in a 200°F oven to keep warm while cooking remaining batches.
Serve waffles warm with desired AIP-friendly toppings like maple syrup, fresh fruit, cinnamon, or coconut butter.

Nutrition per serving (2 waffles without toppings):

Calories: 295
Carbs: 33g
Fiber: 2g
Protein: 6g
Fat: 18g
Notes:

Use very green, unripe plantains for best texture.
Let batter rest 5-10 mins before cooking for fluffier waffles.
Top with AIP breakfast sausage or bacon for added protein.

These grain-free plantain waffles make a delicious, filling breakfast! They have a crispy exterior but stay fluffy and tender on the inside. Easy to make and kid-friendly too.

Cauliflower Breakfast Bowl

Prep Time: 15 minutes
Cook Time: 25 minutes
Total Time: 40 minutes
Servings: 4
Ingredients:

1 medium head cauliflower, cut into florets
2 tbsp avocado oil or olive oil, divided
1 tsp garlic powder
1/2 tsp onion powder
1/4 tsp sea salt
1/4 tsp black pepper
4 cups baby spinach or arugula
2 avocados, diced
4 eggs, cooked to your liking (fried, scrambled, etc.)
AIP-compliant protein of choice (chicken, turkey, salmon), cooked

Instructions:
Preheat oven to 400°F. Line a baking sheet with parchment paper.
In a large bowl, toss the cauliflower florets with 1 tbsp oil, garlic powder, onion powder, salt and pepper until evenly coated.
Spread the cauliflower out in a single layer on the prepared baking sheet. Roast for 20-25 minutes, stirring halfway, until cauliflower is tender and browned.
While cauliflower is roasting, cook your eggs and protein of choice.
To assemble the bowls, place 1 cup of greens in the bottom of each bowl. Top with 1/4 of the roasted cauliflower, 1 cooked egg, 1/4 of the diced avocado, and protein.

Drizzle with remaining 1 tbsp oil or AIP-compliant sauce/dressing if desired.

Nutrition per serving (1 bowl):
Calories: 356
Carbs: 19g
Fiber: 9g
Protein: 17g
Fat: 25g
Notes:

For meal prep, keep components separate and assemble bowls when ready to eat.
Add roasted sweet potatoes, broccoli or other veggies for extra nutrients.
Top with AIP ranch, salsa or chimichurri for extra flavor.

This loaded cauliflower breakfast bowl is nutrient-dense, flavorful and fully AIP-compliant. The garlicky roasted cauliflower pairs perfectly with creamy avocado, greens, eggs and your protein of choice.

AIP Breakfast Casserole

Prep Time: 20 minutes
Cooking Time: 25-30 minutes
Serving Size: 6

Ingredients

1 lb ground beef or turkey, cooked and drained

2 medium sweet potatoes, peeled and thinly sliced

2 cups mixed vegetables (such as bell peppers, onions, and spinach), sautéed

8 eggs (optional, omit if not tolerated)

1 teaspoon dried herbs (such as parsley, thyme, or basil)

Salt and pepper to taste

Cooking Instructions

Set your oven to 375°F (190°C). Grease a baking dish with coconut oil or olive oil. Transfer the cooked ground beef or turkey to the bottom of the dish in an even layer. Top the meat with a layer of thinly sliced sweet potatoes. Finally, cover the sweet potatoes with the sautéed mixed vegetables. Whisk the eggs (if using) with the salt, pepper, and dried herbs in a mixing bowl. Pour the egg mixture evenly over the casserole, covering all the ingredients. Bake in the preheated oven for 25 to 30 minutes, or until the edges are golden brown and the eggs are set. Take the casserole out of the oven and allow it to cool slightly before slicing and serving.

Nutritional Values (per serving):
Calories: 280 kcal, Protein: 20g, Carbs: 15g, Fat: 15g, Fiber: 3, Sugar: 4g

Turmeric Coconut Porridge

Prep Time: 5 minutes
Cooking Time: 15 minutes
Serving Size: 2

Ingredients

2 cups coconut milk

1/2 cup shredded coconut

2 ripe bananas, mashed

1 teaspoon ground turmeric

Sliced bananas and cinnamon for serving

Cooking Instructions

Coconut milk, shredded coconut, mashed bananas, and ground turmeric should all be combined in a saucepan and brought to a gentle simmer over medium-low heat. After that, reduce the heat to low and simmer the porridge, stirring occasionally, until it thickens to the desired consistency, about 10 to 15 minutes. After that, remove the pot from the heat and allow it to cool slightly before serving it warm, garnished with sliced bananas and cinnamon.

Nutritional Values (per serving, without toppings):
Calories: 320 kcal, Protein: 3g, Carbs: 20g, Fat: 27g, Fiber: 5g, Sugar: 12g

Chicken and Vegetable Frittata

Prep Time: 10 minutes
Cooking Time: 20-25 minutes
Serving Size: 4

Ingredients

6 eggs (optional, omit if not tolerated)

1 cup diced cooked chicken

1 cup chopped spinach

1 cup sliced mushrooms

Coconut oil for greasing

Salt and pepper to taste (optional, omit for strict AIP)

Cooking Instructions

Heat a greased skillet over medium heat on the stovetop. Pour the egg mixture into the skillet and spread it evenly. Preheat your oven to 350°F (175°C). In a mixing bowl, beat together the eggs (if using) until well beaten. Stir in diced cooked chicken, chopped spinach, and sliced mushrooms. Season with salt and pepper. (omit for strict AIP). Cook for 3–4 minutes, or until the edges begin to set. Transfer the skillet to the preheated oven and bake for 15-20 minutes, or until the frittata is fully set and slightly golden on top. Remove from the skillet and let cool for a few minutes before slicing; serve with a side of mixed greens.

Nutritional Values (per serving, without optional ingredients):
Calories: 180 kcal, Protein: 20g, Carbs: 3g, Fat: 10g, Fiber: 1g, Sugar: 1g

AIP Breakfast Burrito Bowl

Prep Time: 15 minutes
Cook Time: 25 minutes
Total Time: 40 minutes
Servings: 4
Ingredients:

1 medium head cauliflower, cut into florets
2 tbsp avocado oil or olive oil, divided
1 tsp garlic powder
1/2 tsp onion powder
1/4 tsp sea salt
1/4 tsp black pepper
4 cups baby spinach or arugula
2 avocados, diced
4 eggs, cooked to your liking (fried, scrambled, etc.)
AIP-compliant protein of choice (chicken, turkey, salmon), cooked

Instructions:

Preheat oven to 400°F. Line a baking sheet with parchment paper.
In a large bowl, toss the cauliflower florets with 1 tbsp oil, garlic powder, onion powder, salt and pepper until evenly coated.
Spread the cauliflower out in a single layer on the prepared baking sheet. Roast for 20-25 minutes, stirring halfway, until cauliflower is tender and browned.
While cauliflower is roasting, cook your eggs and protein of choice.

To assemble the bowls, place 1 cup of greens in the bottom of each bowl. Top with 1/4 of the roasted cauliflower, 1 cooked egg, 1/4 of the diced avocado, and protein.

Drizzle with remaining 1 tbsp oil or AIP-compliant sauce/dressing if desired.

Nutrition per serving (1 bowl):
Calories: 356
Carbs: 19g
Fiber: 9g
Protein: 17g
Fat: 25g
Notes:

For meal prep, keep components separate and assemble bowls when ready to eat.

Add roasted sweet potatoes, broccoli or other veggies for extra nutrients.

Top with AIP ranch, salsa or chimichurri for extra flavor.

This loaded cauliflower breakfast bowl is nutrient-dense, flavorful and fully AIP-compliant. The garlicky roasted cauliflower pairs perfectly with creamy avocado, greens, eggs and your protein of choice. Customize it with your favorite AIP-friendly toppings!

Baked Apples with Cinnamon

Prep Time: 10 minutes
Cook Time: 30 minutes
Total Time: 40 minutes
Servings: 4
Ingredients:

4 medium apples (Honeycrisp, Gala or other baking apple)

2 tbsp coconut oil, melted
2 tbsp coconut sugar
1 tsp ground cinnamon
1/4 tsp ground ginger
1/4 tsp ground nutmeg
1 tbsp fresh lemon juice
2 tbsp raisins or dried cranberries (optional)

Instructions:

Preheat oven to 375°F. Grease a baking dish with coconut oil or avocado oil spray.

Core the apples, cutting out most of the inner apple and leaving about 1/2 inch at the bottom intact.

In a small bowl, mix together the melted coconut oil, coconut sugar, cinnamon, ginger, nutmeg and lemon juice.

Stuff each apple cavity evenly with the coconut oil/sugar mixture. Place stuffed apples in the prepared baking dish.

If using raisins or cranberries, sprinkle them evenly over the tops of the apples.

Pour 1/4 cup of water into the bottom of the baking dish.

Bake for 25-30 minutes, until apples are fork-tender and filling is bubbling.

Allow to cool slightly before serving warm. Can be topped with coconut cream or AIP granola, if desired.

Nutrition per serving (1 stuffed baked apple without toppings):
Calories: 158
Carbs: 27g
Fiber: 4g
Protein: 1g
Fat: 6g

These warm, cinnamon-spiced baked apples are a cozy breakfast or brunch treat! They are naturally sweetened with coconut sugar and filled with a gingery cinnamon filling. Easy to make and customize with your favorite dried fruits and toppings. Enjoy them as a nutrient-dense start to your day while following the AIP diet.

Chapter 2: AIP Snacks and Sweets AIP Recipes

Baked Sweet Potato Chips

Prep Time: 10 minutes
Cooking Time: 20-25 minutes
Serving Size: 4

Ingredients

2 medium sweet potatoes, thinly sliced

2 tablespoons coconut oil, melted

Sea salt to taste

Cooking Instructions

Set aside a baking sheet lined with parchment paper, preheat your oven to 375°F (190°C), wash and peel your sweet potatoes, and then use a mandoline slicer or a sharp knife to thinly slice them into rounds. Transfer the sliced sweet potatoes to a large bowl and toss them with melted coconut oil until well coated. Arrange your sweet potato slices in a single layer, being careful not to overlap, on the prepared baking sheet. Dredge the sweet potato slices in sea salt; bake in the preheated oven for 20 to 25 minutes, rotating the chips halfway through, until they become crispy and golden brown. Take the chips out of the oven and allow them to cool for a short while before serving.

Nutritional Values (per serving):
Calories: 120 kcal, Protein: 1g, Carbs: 15g, Fat: 7, Fiber: 2g, Sugar: 3g

Coconut Berry Bliss Balls

Prep Time: 10 minutes
Serving Size: 12 bliss balls

Ingredients

1 cup unsweetened shredded coconut

1/2 cup mixed berries (such as strawberries, blueberries, or raspberries), fresh or thawed if frozen

1/4 cup coconut butter

1 tablespoon honey (optional, omit if not tolerated)

1/2 teaspoon vanilla extract (optional, omit if not tolerated)

Pinch of sea salt

Cooking Instructions

Shredded coconut, mixed berries, coconut butter, honey, vanilla extract, and a small pinch of sea salt should all be combined in a food processor and pulsed until a thick dough forms. Using your hands, roll the dough into small balls that are about 1 inch in diameter. To firm up, place the bliss balls on a baking sheet lined with parchment paper and refrigerate for at least half an hour. Once firm, store the bliss balls in the refrigerator in an airtight container until you're ready to serve.

Nutritional Values (per serving, based on 1 bliss ball):
Calories: 70 kcal, Protein: 1g, Carbs: 5g, Fat: 6g, Fiber: 2g, Sugar: 3g

Cucumber Avocado Boats

Prep Time: 10 minutes
Serving Size: 4

Ingredients

2 large cucumbers

1 ripe avocado

1/2 lemon, juiced

1/4 cup diced red bell pepper

1/4 cup diced cucumber (from the scooped out center)

1 tablespoon chopped fresh cilantro

Salt to taste

Cooking Instructions

Slice the cucumbers lengthwise in half, then remove the seeds to form "boats". In a bowl, mash the avocado with the lemon juice until it becomes smooth. Add the diced red bell pepper, diced cucumber, chopped cilantro, and salt to taste. Evenly fill each cucumber boat with the avocado mixture.

Nutritional Values (per serving):
Calories: 90 kcal, Protein: 2g, Carbs: 7g, Fat: 7g, Fiber: 4g, Sugar: 2g

AIP Trail Mix

Prep Time: 5 minutes
Serving Size: 8

Ingredients

1 cup unsweetened coconut flakes

1/2 cup sliced or chopped dried fruit (such as unsweetened dried mango, apple, or banana)

1/2 cup raw pumpkin seeds (pepitas)

1/2 cup raw sunflower seeds

1/4 cup dried cranberries (look for ones sweetened with apple juice or omit if preferred)

1/4 cup raw or lightly toasted coconut chips

1/4 teaspoon sea salt

Cooking Instructions

To ensure even distribution of ingredients, combine all the ingredients in a large mixing bowl and toss well. Store the trail mix in an airtight container until you're ready to serve it or pack it for snacks.

Nutritional Values (per serving, approximately 1/4 cup):
Calories: 180 kcal, Protein: 4g, Carbs: 15g, Fat: 12g, Fiber: 4g, Sugar: 8g

Baked Cinnamon Apples

Prep Time: 10 minutes
Cooking Time: 35–40 minutes
Serving Size: 4

Ingredients

4 medium-sized apples, cored and sliced

1 teaspoon ground cinnamon

1 tablespoon coconut oil, melted

1 tablespoon honey or maple syrup (optional, omit for strict AIP)

1/4 cup water

Cooking Instructions

Set the oven to 350°F (175°C). In a bowl, combine the sliced apples, melted coconut oil, ground cinnamon, and honey or maple syrup (if desired). Make sure the apples are well coated. Transfer the apple slices to a baking dish and cover the apples with water. Place aluminum foil over the baking dish and bake in the preheated oven for 25 to 30 minutes, stirring the apples halfway through. After that, take off the foil and bake for a further 5 to 10 minutes to allow the liquid to slightly reduce.

Nutritional Values (per serving):
Calories: 100 kcal, Protein: 0g, Carbs: 25g, Fat: 3g, Fiber: 4g, Sugar: 19g

Chapter 3: AIP Vegetarian and Vegan AIP Recipes

Roasted Sweet Potato and Kale Salad

Prep Time: 10 minutes
Cooking Time: 25 minutes
Serving Size: 4

Ingredients

2 medium sweet potatoes, peeled and cubed

4 cups kale, stems removed and torn into bite-sized pieces

2 tablespoons olive oil

Salt to taste

For the Lemon-Tahini Dressing:

1/4 cup tahini

2 tablespoons lemon juice

1 tablespoon apple cider vinegar

1 clove garlic, minced

2-3 tablespoons water (adjust for desired consistency)

Salt to taste

Cooking Instructions

Set the oven to 400°F (200°C). Take a baking sheet, add some olive oil, sprinkle some salt on it, and toss to coat it evenly. Roast the sweet potatoes for 20 to 25 minutes, or until they are soft and lightly browned, turning them over halfway through. In the meantime, prepare the kale by putting it in a big bowl, drizzling it with some olive oil and salt, and massaging it with your hands for a few minutes until it softens. Whisk together the tahini, lemon juice, apple cider vinegar, minced garlic, and water in a small bowl until smooth. Season with salt to taste. When the sweet potatoes are done roasting, let them cool slightly. To assemble the salad, place the massaged kale in a serving bowl or platter, top with the roasted sweet potatoes, and drizzle with the lemon-tahini dressing.

Nutritional Values (per serving):
Calories: 250 kcal, Protein: 5g, Carbs: 25g, Fat: 15g, Fiber: 5g, Sugar: 4g

Cauliflower Rice Stir-Fry

Prep Time: 10 minutes
Cooking Time: 15 minutes
Serving Size: 4

Ingredients

1 head cauliflower, riced (or 4 cups pre-riced cauliflower)

1 bell pepper, thinly sliced

1 carrot, thinly sliced

1 cup broccoli florets

2 tablespoons coconut aminos

2 cloves garlic, minced

2 tablespoons coconut oil

Salt to taste

Optional: chopped green onions for garnish

Cooking Instructions

In a big skillet or wok over medium heat, heat the coconut oil. Add the minced garlic and sauté for about 1 minute until fragrant. Add the bell pepper, carrot, and broccoli florets, and stir-fry for about 5-7 minutes, or until the vegetables are soft and crisp.

Add the riced cauliflower and cook, stirring frequently, for an additional 3–4 minutes, or until the cauliflower is cooked through but still slightly firm. Add coconut aminos to the cauliflower rice and vegetable mixture, stir to mix, and cook for an additional two to three minutes to let the flavors meld. Taste and adjust the seasoning. Take off the heat and serve hot, topped with finely chopped green onions.

Nutritional Values (per serving):
Calories: 100 kcal, Protein: 3g, Carbs: 12g, Fat: 6g, Fiber: 4g, Sugar: 5g

Noodles with Pesto

Prep Time: 15 minutes
Cooking Time: 5 minutes
Serving Size: 4

Ingredients

4 medium zucchinis, spiralized into noodles

1 ripe avocado

1 cup fresh basil leaves

2 cloves garlic, minced

2 tablespoons olive oil

Salt to taste

Optional toppings: chopped fresh tomatoes, sliced black olives, pine nuts (if tolerated)

Cooking Instructions

To make the avocado pesto, place the avocado, minced garlic, basil leaves, olive oil, and a small pinch of salt in a blender or food processor and process until smooth and creamy. In a large skillet, heat a small amount of olive oil over medium heat. Add the zucchini noodles and cook, tossing occasionally, for two to three minutes, or until they are soft but still have a slight crunch. After the zucchini noodles are cooked, take them off the heat and place them in a serving bowl.

Drizzle the avocado pesto over the noodles and toss to coat them thoroughly. If preferred, garnish the dish with additional toppings.

Nutritional Values (per serving, without optional toppings):
Calories: 150 kcal, Protein: 3g, Carbs: 10g, Fat: 12g, Fiber: 5g, Sugar: 4g

Portobello Mushroom Burgers

Prep Time: 10 minutes
Cooking Time: 10-14 minutes
Serving Size: 4

Ingredients

4 large portobello mushrooms, stems removed

1 avocado, sliced

1 roasted red pepper, sliced

4 large lettuce leaves

Salt to taste

Optional: AIP-friendly sauce (e.g., homemade olive oil and lemon dressing)

Cooking Instructions

Turn the heat up to medium-high. Wipe off any dirt from the portobello mushrooms with a damp cloth. Drizzle both sides with a little olive oil and season with salt. Put the mushrooms, gill-side down, on the grill and cook for 5 to 7 minutes on each side, or until they are soft and have grill marks. Prepare the lettuce leaves on serving plates while the mushrooms are grilling. When the mushrooms are done, place them on top of the lettuce leaves. Garnish each mushroom with sliced avocado and roasted red peppers. Serve, with the option to drizzle with sauce that is suitable for the AIP.

Nutritional Values (per serving):
Calories: 100 kcal, Protein: 3g, Carbs: 8g, Fat: 7g, Fiber: 4g, Sugar: 2g

Stuffed Bell Peppers

Prep Time: 15 minutes
Cooking Time: 40-45 minutes
Serving Size: 4 servings

Ingredients

4 large bell peppers (any color), halved and seeds removed

2 cups cauliflower rice

1 cup cooked lentils or chickpeas (if tolerated)

1 small onion, diced

2 cloves garlic, minced

1 tablespoon coconut oil

1 teaspoon dried oregano

1 teaspoon dried basil

Salt to taste

Fresh parsley, chopped (for garnish)

Cooking Instructions

A large skillet should be heated to 375°F (190°C). In the skillet, add the minced garlic and diced onion and sauté for 3–4 minutes, or until the onion is softened. Next, add the cauliflower rice and cook for another 5–7 minutes, or until it is tender. Finally, add the cooked lentils or chickpeas, dried oregano, dried basil, and salt to taste.

Cook for a further 2–3 minutes, or until the flavors meld. Lay out the cut side up bell pepper halves in a baking dish. Spoon the cauliflower rice mixture into each half, gently pressing to pack it in. Cover the baking dish with foil and bake in the preheated oven for 25 to 30 minutes, or until the bell peppers are soft. Then, take off the foil and bake for a further 5 to 10 minutes to lightly brown the tops. Before serving, garnish with fresh parsley that has been chopped.

Nutritional Values (per serving):
Calories: 220 kcal, Protein: 10g, Carbs: 30g, Fat: 6g, Fiber: 10g, Sugar: 10g

Butternut Squash Soup

Prep Time: 15 minutes
Cooking Time: 25 minutes
Serving Size: 4

Ingredients

1 medium butternut squash, peeled, seeded, and diced

1 can (13.5 oz) coconut milk

1 tablespoon fresh ginger, grated

1 teaspoon ground turmeric

4 cups bone broth or vegetable broth

Salt to taste

Fresh herbs (such as parsley or cilantro) for garnish

Cooking Instructions

Diced butternut squash, coconut milk, grated ginger, ground turmeric, and broth should all be combined in a large pot. Heat the mixture to a boil over medium-high heat, then lower the heat and simmer until the butternut squash is tender, about 20 to 25 minutes. Puree the soup with an immersion blender or regular blender until it's smooth and creamy, and then serve hot, garnished with fresh herbs.

Nutritional Values (per serving):
Calories: 220 kcal, Protein: 4g, Carbs: 25g, Fat: 14, Fiber: 5g, Sugar: 6g

Crispy Baked Plantain Chips

Prep Time: 10 minutes
Cooking Time: 15-20 minutes
Serving Size: 4

Ingredients

2 green plantains

2 tablespoons coconut oil, melted

Sea salt to taste

Guacamole or salsa for serving (optional)

Cooking Instructions

Set aside a large bowl, toss the plantain slices with melted coconut oil until evenly coated, then arrange the slices in a single layer, making sure they are not overlapping, on the prepared baking sheet. Preheat your oven to 375°F (190°C). Peel and thinly slice the plantains using a sharp knife or mandoline slicer. Sprinkle the plantain slices with sea salt to taste. Bake in the preheated oven for 15-20 minutes, flipping halfway through. When the plantain chips are crispy and golden brown, remove from the oven and allow to cool for a few minutes before serving. You can serve the crispy baked plantain chips with salsa or guacamole, if you'd like.

Nutritional Values (per serving, without dip):
Calories: 120 kcal, Protein: 1g, Carbs: 20g, Fat: 5g, Fiber: 2g, Sugar: 8g

Cabbage Rolls with Cauliflower Rice

Prep Time: 30 minutes
Cooking Time: 50 minutes
Serving Size: 4

Ingredients

1 head of cabbage

1 small head of cauliflower

1 cup mushrooms, finely chopped

1 small onion, finely chopped

2 cloves garlic, minced

1 teaspoon dried thyme

1 teaspoon dried oregano

Salt to taste

1 can (14 oz) AIP-friendly tomato sauce

1 cup bone broth or water

Fresh parsley, chopped (for garnish)

Cooking Instructions

Cut the cauliflower into florets and pulse in a food processor until it resembles rice. Preheat the oven to 350°F (175°C). Bring a large pot of water to a boil. Carefully remove the outer leaves of the cabbage and blanch them in the boiling water for two to three minutes, until softened. Set aside to cool.

Add the chopped onions, garlic, and mushrooms to a skillet over medium heat. Cook until the ingredients soften, about 5 minutes. Add the cauliflower "rice" to the skillet and cook for an additional 5 minutes. Stir in the dried oregano and dried thyme, and adjust with salt to taste. Take the skillet off the heat. Spoon a spoonful of the cauliflower mixture onto each cabbage leaf. Roll the cabbage leaf up, tucking in the sides as you roll. Place seam side down in a baking dish. After combining the tomato sauce, bone broth, or water in a bowl, pour the mixture over the cabbage rolls in the baking dish, cover with aluminum foil, and bake in the preheated oven for 45 to 50 minutes, or until the rolls are tender. Before serving, sprinkle the rolls with chopped parsley.

Nutritional Values (per serving):
Calories: 180 kcal, Protein: 6g, Carbs: 25g, Fat: 6g, Fiber: 9g, Sugar: 12g

Coconut Curry Veggie Stir-Fry

Prep Time: 10 minutes
Cooking Time: 15 minutes
Serving Size: 4

Ingredients

2 tablespoons coconut oil

4 cups mixed vegetables (such as bell peppers, broccoli, carrots, snap peas)

2 cloves garlic, minced

1 teaspoon minced ginger

1 teaspoon curry powder (AIP-friendly blend)

1/2 teaspoon turmeric powder

1/2 cup coconut milk

Salt to taste

Fresh cilantro for garnish (optional)

Cooking Instructions

In a large skillet or wok over medium heat, heat the coconut oil. Add the minced garlic and ginger and sauté for 1 minute, or until fragrant. Add the mixed vegetables to the skillet and stir-fry for 5 to 7 minutes, or until they are crisp-tender.

Sprinkle the vegetables with curry powder and turmeric powder and stir to coat them evenly. After adding the coconut milk to the skillet and thoroughly mixing, cook the vegetables for two to three more minutes, or until they are heated through. Season with salt and, if preferred, garnish with fresh cilantro.

Nutritional Values (per serving):
Calories: 120 kcal, Protein: 2g, Carbs: 10g, Fat: 9g, Fiber: 3g, Sugar: 4g

Baked Acorn Squash with Cinnamon

Prep Time: 10 minutes
Cooking Time: 35-50 minutes
Serving Size: 4

Ingredients

2 acorn squash, halved and seeds removed

Cinnamon (AIP-friendly)

Cooking Instructions

After preheating the oven to 400°F (200°C), place the cut side down acorn squash halves on a baking sheet lined with parchment paper. Bake the squash for 30 to 40 minutes, or until it is tender and pierces easily with a fork. Once the squash is done, remove it from the oven and carefully turn it over so the cut side is now facing up. Scatter the exposed flesh of the squash with the cinnamon, then return it to the oven and bake for a further 5 to 10 minutes, letting the cinnamon seep into the squash. After that, take it out of the oven and allow it to cool slightly before serving.

Nutritional Values (per serving):
Calories: 80 kcal, Protein: 1g, Carbs: 20g, Fat: 0g, Fiber: 4g, Sugar: 0g

Mashed Turnips with Herbs

Prep Time: 10 minutes
Cooking Time: 20 minutes
Serving Size: 4

Ingredients

4 medium turnips, peeled and diced

2 cloves garlic, minced

1/4 cup coconut milk

2 tablespoons fresh parsley or chives, chopped

Salt to taste

Cooking Instructions

Turnips should be diced and placed in a pot with water to cover. Turnips should be brought to a boil over medium-high heat, then simmered for 15 to 20 minutes, or until fork-tender. Once the turnips are cooked, they should be drained and put back in the pot along with chopped fresh herbs, minced garlic, and coconut milk. Mash the turnips with a potato masher or fork until the desired consistency is reached. Add a little more coconut milk if the mixture is too thick. Season to taste and stir to combine. Serve hot, garnished with extra fresh herbs.

Nutritional Values (per serving):
Calories: 70 kcal, Protein: 2g, Carbs: 10g, Fat: 3g, Fiber: 3g, Sugar: 5g

Grilled Eggplant with Balsamic Glaze

Prep Time: 10 minutes
Cooking Time: 10–15 minutes
Serving Size: 4

Ingredients

1 large eggplant, sliced into rounds

2 tablespoons extra virgin olive oil

Salt to taste

1/2 cup balsamic vinegar

Fresh basil leaves for garnish

Cooking Instructions

Preheat the grill to medium-high heat. Brush the eggplant slices on both sides with olive oil and season with salt. Grill the eggplant slices for 3–4 minutes on each side, or until they are soft and caramelized; depending on the size of your grill, you may need to cook them in batches. While the eggplant is grilling, make the balsamic glaze. In a small saucepan, bring the vinegar to a simmer over medium heat. Cook for 5-7 minutes, stirring occasionally, until the vinegar has reduced by half and has a syrupy consistency. When the eggplant is perfectly grilled, remove it from the grill and place it on a serving platter. Drizzle the grilled eggplant slices with the balsamic glaze. Garnish with fresh basil leaves.

Nutritional Values (per serving):
Calories: 90 kcal, Protein: 1g, Carbs: 12g, Fat: 4g, Fiber: 4g, Sugar: 7g

Cauliflower Mashed Potatoes

Prep Time: 10 minutes
Cooking Time: 10 minutes
Serving Size: 4

Ingredients

1 medium head of cauliflower, chopped into florets

1/4 cup coconut milk

2 cloves garlic, minced

2 tablespoons nutritional yeast

Salt to taste

Cooking Instructions

Steam the cauliflower until the florets are tender, 8 to 10 minutes. Then, transfer the steamed cauliflower to a food processor or blender. Add the coconut milk, nutritional yeast, minced garlic, and a pinch of salt. Blend until smooth and creamy, adding more coconut milk to reach the desired consistency. Taste and adjust the seasoning. Serve hot as a tasty and healthy substitute for mashed potatoes.

Nutritional Values (per serving):
Calories: 70 kcal, Protein: 3g, Carbs: 9g, Fat: 3g, Fiber: 4g, Sugar: 3g

Spinach and Mushroom Avocado Dressing

Prep Time: 10 minutes
Serving Size: 4

Ingredients

6 cups fresh spinach leaves

1 cup sliced mushrooms

1 ripe avocado

2 tablespoons fresh lemon juice

2 tablespoons extra virgin olive oil

Salt to taste

Optional toppings: sliced radishes, shredded carrots, or diced cucumber

Cooking Instructions

Fresh spinach leaves and sliced mushrooms should be combined in a large mixing bowl. In a small bowl, mash the ripe avocado with a fork until smooth. Add fresh lemon juice, extra virgin olive oil, and a pinch of salt to the mashed avocado, and mix until well combined to make the dressing. Pour the avocado dressing over the spinach and mushroom mixture, tossing gently to coat the salad evenly.

Divide the salad onto serving plates, and garnish with desired toppings.

Nutritional Values (per serving):
Calories: 150 kcal, Protein: 3g, Carbs: 9g, Fat: 12g, Fiber: 5g, Sugar: 1g

Stuffed Acorn Squash and Cranberries

Prep Time: 15 minutes
Cooking Time: 40-45 minutes
Serving Size: 4

Ingredients

2 acorn squash, halved and seeds removed

1 cup cooked quinoa

1/2 cup dried cranberries

1/4 cup chopped nuts (such as walnuts or pecans)

2 tablespoons chopped fresh herbs (such as parsley or thyme)

Salt to taste

Coconut oil for roasting

Cooking Instructions

Heat the oven to 400°F (200°C). Coat the insides of the acorn squash halves with coconut oil and season with salt. Lay the halves, cut side down, on a baking sheet covered with parchment paper. Roast in the oven for 25 to 30 minutes, or until they are soft. Transfer the cooked quinoa, chopped nuts, dried cranberries, and fresh herbs into a mixing bowl. Adjust the seasoning with salt. When the squash halves are soft, take them out of the oven and carefully turn them over. Spoon the quinoa mixture into each half, making sure to pack it in tightly.

Place the filled squash halves back into the oven and bake for a further ten to fifteen minutes, or until they are thoroughly heated and have a crunchy top.

Nutritional Values (per serving):
Calories: 250 kcal, Protein: 5g, Carbs: 45g, Fat: 7g, Fiber: 7g, Sugar: 10g

Chapter 4: AIP Poultry, Meat and Potatoes AIP Recipes

Chicken Breast

Prep Time: 5 minutes
Cooking Time: 12-25 minutes
Serving Size: 4

Ingredients

4 boneless, skinless chicken breasts

2 tablespoons coconut oil or olive oil

Salt to taste

AIP-friendly herbs and spices (e.g., garlic powder, onion powder, dried thyme)

Cooking Instructions

To ensure that your chicken breasts don't stick, brush them with oil before grilling them for 6-7 minutes on each side, or until they reach an internal temperature of 165°F (75°C). If you're using an oven, skillet, or grill, preheat the heat to medium-high. Pat the chicken breasts dry with paper towels and season both sides with salt and AIP-friendly herbs and spices. To bake: Preheat your oven to 400°F (200°C). Arrange the seasoned chicken breasts on a baking sheet lined with parchment paper. Bake for 20 to 25 minutes, or until the chicken reaches an internal temperature of 165°F (75°C). Alternatively, you can sauté the chicken by heating coconut oil or olive oil in a skillet over medium-high heat.

After the chicken is cooked through and has a golden brown exterior, remove it from the heat source.

Nutritional Values (per serving 4 oz cooked chicken breast):
Calories: 150 kca, Protein: 30g, Fat: 3g, Sodium: 60mg

Turkey Thighs

Prep Time: 10 minutes
Cooking Time: 1½to 2 hours
Serving Size: 4

Ingredients

4 turkey thighs, bone-in and skin removed

2 tablespoons coconut oil

2 teaspoons dried thyme

2 teaspoons dried oregano

2 teaspoons garlic powder

Salt to taste

1 cup chicken or turkey broth

Cooking Instructions

In a small bowl, combine the dried thyme, dried oregano, garlic powder, and salt. Rub the spice mixture evenly over the turkey thighs. Preheat your oven to 325°F (163°C). Warm up the coconut oil in a large skillet over medium-high heat. Add the turkey thighs to the skillet and brown on both sides, about 3–4 minutes per side. Transfer the browned turkey thighs to a baking dish. Fill the baking dish with chicken or turkey broth, cover with aluminum foil, and pop into the preheated oven. Bake the turkey thighs for one and a half to two hours, or until they are tender and cooked through.

Take the baking dish out of the oven and allow the turkey thighs to rest for a few minutes before serving.

Duck Breast

Prep Time: 5 minutes
Cooking Time: 10-12 minutes
Serving Size: 2

Ingredients

2 duck breasts

Salt to taste

AIP-friendly herbs and spices (such as thyme, rosemary, and garlic powder)

Cooking Instructions

Preheat a skillet over medium-high heat. Score the duck breasts' skin in a crisscross pattern, being careful not to cut into the meat. Season the duck breasts on both sides with salt and your preferred AIP-friendly herbs and spices. Place the duck breasts skin-side down in the skillet and cook for 5 to 7 minutes, until the skin is golden brown and crispy. After a few minutes, turn the duck breasts over and cook for a further three to five minutes, or until done to your liking. Take the duck breasts out of the skillet and allow them to cool before slicing.

Nutritional Values (per serving):
Calories: 250 kcal, Protein: 20g, Carbs: 0g, Fat: 18g, Fiber: 0g, Sugar: 0g

Cornish Hen

Prep Time: 10 minutes
Cooking Time: 60-75 minutes
Serving Size: 2 servings

Ingredients

2 Cornish hens

2 tablespoons coconut oil, melted

2 teaspoons dried thyme

2 teaspoons dried oregano

2 teaspoons garlic powder

Salt to taste

Cooking Instructions

Preheat the oven to 375°F (190°C). Rinse the hens under cold water and pat dry with paper towels. In a small bowl, combine the melted coconut oil, dried thyme, dried oregano, garlic powder, and salt. Rub the herb mixture all over the hens, making sure to coat them evenly. A roasting pan or baking dish should be used for the Cornish hens. Roast in the preheated oven for approximately 60–75 minutes, or until the internal temperature reaches 165°F (74°C) when measured with a meat thermometer inserted into the thickest part of the hen. Once cooked, remove the Cornish hens from the oven and allow them to rest for 5–10 minutes before serving.

Nutritional Values (per serving):
Calories: 400 kcal, Protein: 40g, Carbs: 0g, Fat: 26g, Fiber: 0g, Sugar: 0g

Quail

Prep Time: 10 minutes
Cooking Time: 25–30 minutes
Serving Size: 4

Ingredients

4 whole quails, cleaned

2 tablespoons coconut oil

2 cloves garlic, minced

1 teaspoon dried thyme

Salt to taste

Cooking Instructions

Set the oven to 375°F (190°C). Combine the minced garlic, dried thyme, and salt in a small bowl. Apply coconut oil to the quails, then evenly coat them with the herb mixture. Transfer the quails to an oven-safe skillet or roasting pan. Roast in the preheated oven for 25 to 30 minutes, or until the quails are cooked through and golden brown, basting them occasionally with the pan juices. Remove from the oven and let the quails rest for a few minutes before serving.

Nutritional Values (per serving):
Calories: 180 kcal, Protein: 25g, Carbs: 0g, Fat: 8g, Cholesterol: 95mg, Sodium: 65mg

Beef Chuck Roast

Prep Time: 15 minutes
Cooking Time: 2½ –3 hours
Serving Size: 4–6

Ingredients

2-3 lbs beef chuck roast

2 tablespoons coconut oil or olive oil

1 onion, sliced

3 cloves garlic, minced

2 carrots, chopped

2 celery stalks, chopped

1 cup bone broth or beef broth (check for AIP-compliant ingredients)

2 bay leaves

1 teaspoon dried thyme

Salt to taste

Cooking Instructions

Preheat your oven to 325°F (160°C). In a Dutch oven or oven-safe pot, heat up some coconut oil or olive oil over medium-high heat. Sear the beef chuck roast on all sides until browned, about 3-4 minutes per side. Remove the roast from the pot and set aside. Add the chopped onion, minced garlic, chopped carrots, and chopped celery, and cook for 5 to 7 minutes, or until the vegetables begin to soften.

Return the roast to the pot, add the bone broth or beef broth, bay leaves, dried thyme, and salt to taste. Cover the pot with a lid and place it in the preheated oven; cook for 2.5 to 3 hours, or until the beef is tender and easily pulls apart with a fork. Once cooked, remove the pot from the oven and let it rest for a few minutes before serving. Serve the beef chuck roast hot, sliced or shredded, with the vegetables and juices from the pot.

Nutritional Values (per serving):
Calories: 350 kcal, Protein: 30g, Carbs: 6g, Fat: 23g, Fiber: 1g, Sugar: 2g

Lamb Chops

Prep Time: 5 minutes
Cooking Time: 8-10 minutes
Serving Size: 2

Ingredients

4 lamb chops

2 tablespoons coconut oil

2 cloves garlic, minced (optional, omit if sensitive)

1 teaspoon dried rosemary

1 teaspoon dried thyme

Salt to taste

Cooking Instructions

Combine salt, dried thyme, and rosemary in a small bowl. Apply the herb mixture evenly to the lamb chops on both sides. Heat coconut oil in a skillet over medium-high heat. Add the lamb chops and sear for 3–4 minutes on each side, or until done to your liking. Remove the lamb chops from the skillet and let rest for a few minutes before serving; if using minced garlic, add it to the skillet during the last minute of cooking, stirring constantly to avoid burning.

Nutritional Values (per serving):
Calories: 300 kcal, Protein: 22g, Carbs: 0g, Fat: 23g, Fiber: 0g, Sugar: 0g

Pork Tenderloin

Prep Time: 10 minutes (plus marinating time)
Cooking Time: 25-30 minutes
Serving Size: 4

Ingredients

1 lb pork tenderloin

2 tablespoons apple cider vinegar

2 tablespoons coconut aminos

2 cloves garlic, minced

1 teaspoon dried thyme

1 teaspoon dried rosemary

1/2 teaspoon sea salt

1/4 teaspoon black pepper (optional, omit for strict AIP)

Cooking Instructions

Whisk together the coconut aminos, minced garlic, dried thyme, dried rosemary, sea salt, and black pepper in a small bowl. Transfer the pork tenderloin to a shallow dish or resealable plastic bag, making sure the tenderloin is well coated with the marinade. Marinate for a minimum of 30 minutes, or up to 4 hours, for the most flavor. Set your oven to 400°F (200°C).

Take the pork tenderloin out of the marinade and throw away any extra marinade. Transfer the pork tenderloin to a baking dish or a parchment paper-lined baking sheet. Roast the pork tenderloin for 25 to 30 minutes, rotating it halfway through, or until the internal temperature reaches 145°F (63°C). After cooking, take the pork tenderloin out of the oven and allow it to rest for 5 minutes before slicing.

Nutritional Values (per serving):
Calories: 180 kcal, Protein: 25g, Carbs: 2g, Fat: 7g, Fiber: 0g, Sugar: 0g

Venison

Prep Time: 10 minutes
Cooking Time: 20-25 minutes
Serving Size: 4

Ingredients

1 lb venison, preferably a tender cut like loin or tenderloin

2 tablespoons coconut oil or avocado oil

2 cloves garlic, minced (optional, omit if sensitive)

1 teaspoon dried thyme

1 teaspoon dried rosemary

Salt to taste

Cooking Instructions

Pat the venison dry with paper towels and season generously with salt. In a small bowl, combine the coconut oil or avocado oil, minced garlic, dried thyme, and dried rosemary to make a seasoning mixture. Rub the seasoning mixture all over the venison, making sure it's evenly coated. Preheat your oven to 375°F (190°C). In a roasting pan or oven-safe skillet, place the seasoned venison. Roast in the preheated oven for about 20 to 25 minutes for medium-rare, or until an internal meat thermometer reads 135°F (57°C). After taking the venison out of the oven, let it rest for 5 to 10 minutes before slicing. Serve the venison hot, thinly sliced against the grain.

Nutritional Values (per serving):
Calories: 180 kcal, Protein: 25g, Carbs: 0g, Fat: 9g, Fiber: 0g, Sugar: 0g

Buffalo/Bison

Prep Time: 10 minutes
Cooking Time: 15 minutes
Serving Size: 4

Ingredients

1 lb bison meat, thinly sliced

2 tablespoons coconut oil

3 cloves garlic, minced

1 tablespoon grated ginger

2 cups sliced vegetables (such as bell peppers, carrots, and broccoli)

2 tablespoons coconut aminos

Salt to taste

Optional: chopped green onions for garnish

Cooking Instructions

Heat the coconut oil in a large skillet or wok over medium-high heat. Add the grated ginger and minced garlic and cook for 1 to 2 minutes until fragrant. Cook the bison meat thinly sliced for 2 to 3 minutes until browned. Add the sliced vegetables and stir-fry for 5 to 7 minutes, or until they begin to soften. Add the coconut aminos to the stir-fry and cook for an additional two to three minutes, or until everything is well combined and heated through.

Taste and add salt as needed. You can also garnish with chopped green onions if you like.

Nutritional Values (per serving):
Calories: 250 kcal, Protein: 25g, Carbs: 8g, Fat: 13g, Fiber: 2g, Sugar: 3g

Sweet Potatoes

Prep Time: 10 minutes
Cooking Time: 25-30 minutes
Serving Size: 4

Ingredients

4 medium sweet potatoes

2 tablespoons coconut oil, melted

Salt to taste

Optional: AIP-friendly herbs or spices like garlic powder, onion powder, or thyme

Cooking Instructions

Set the oven to 400°F (200°C). Scrub and wash the sweet potatoes under running water to get rid of any dirt. Peel and cut the sweet potatoes into cubes or wedges, depending on your choice. Transfer the sweet potatoes to a big mixing bowl and coat them evenly with melted coconut oil. Season with salt and any optional AIP-friendly herbs or spices. Spread the sweet potatoes in a single layer on a baking sheet lined with parchment paper or aluminum foil. Roast in the preheated oven for 25 to 30 minutes, or until the sweet potatoes are tender and lightly browned, flipping halfway through cooking. Once cooked, remove from the oven and let cool slightly before serving.

Nutritional Values (per serving):
Calories: 150 kcal, Protein: 2g, Carbs: 26g, Fat: 5g, Fiber: 4g, Sugar: 6g

Japanese Sweet Potatoes

Prep Time: 5 minutes
Cooking Time: 45-60 minutes
Serving Size: 4

Ingredients

4 Japanese sweet potatoes

Cooking Instructions

Set the oven to 400°F (200°C). Rinse and pat dry the Japanese sweet potatoes. Prick each one several times with a fork to release steam while cooking. Transfer the potatoes to a baking sheet covered with aluminum foil or parchment paper. Bake the sweet potatoes in the preheated oven for 45 to 60 minutes, or until a fork inserted into them pierces them easily.

Nutritional Values (per serving):
Calories: 130 kcal, Protein: 2g, Carbs: 30g, Fat: 0g, Fiber: 4g, Sugar: 6g

White Potatoes

Prep Time: 10 minutes
Cooking Time: 15-20 minutes
Serving Size: 4

Ingredients

4 medium-sized white potatoes, peeled and cubed

Water for boiling

Salt (optional)

Cooking Instructions

After peeling and chopping the white potatoes into uniform-sized cubes, put the cubed potatoes in a big pot with water, and if you want, add a pinch of salt. Bring the water to a boil over high heat, then lower the heat to medium-low and simmer the potatoes until they are tender, about 15 to 20 minutes. After that time, drain the potatoes in a colander. When it comes to potatoes, they can be served hot as a side dish or used as a foundation for other AIP-friendly toppings or sauces. For mashed potatoes, drain the potatoes and place them in a mixing bowl. Use a fork or potato masher to mash the potatoes until they're smooth. If you want to make them extra creamy, you can add a little bit of coconut milk or olive oil.

Nutritional Values (per serving, boiled potatoes):
Calories: 100 kcal, Protein: 2g, Carbs: 23g, Fat: 0g, Fiber: 2g, Sugar: 1g

Nutritional Values (per serving, mashed potatoes):
Calories: 120 kcal, Protein: 2g, Carbs: 26g, Fat: 1g, Fiber: 3g, Sugar: 1g

Yuca

Prep Time: 10 minutes
Cooking Time: 20-30 minutes
Serving Size: 4

Ingredients

1 large yuca root (cassava)

Water for boiling

Salt to taste

Cooking Instructions

After removing any tough or woody parts from the yuca root, peel it and cut it into chunks or slices. Rinse the yuca pieces under cold water to get rid of any dirt or debris. Bring a pot of salted water to a boil over high heat, add the yuca pieces, and cook for 20 to 30 minutes, or until the yuca is fork-tender. Once cooked, drain and transfer to a serving dish. You can mash or fry the yuca for a creamy or crispy texture, or serve hot as a side dish.

Nutritional Values (per serving, boiled yuca):
Calories: 220 kcal, Carbs: 55g, Fiber: 3g, Protein: 2g, Fat: 0g, Vitamin C: 42mg, Potassium: 558mg

Boiled Taro Root

Prep Time: 10 minutes
Cooking Time: 20-25 minutes
Serving Size: 4

Ingredients

2 medium taro roots

Water

Salt (optional)

Cooking Instructions

After peeling and cutting the taro roots into chunks or cubes, put the pieces in a pot with water, and optionally add a pinch of salt. Bring the water to a boil, then lower the heat and simmer the taro roots until they are soft to the touch when pierced with a fork. Once the taro roots are cooked, drain them and serve hot as a side dish or use them in other AIP recipes.

Nutritional Values (per serving):
Calories: 160 kcal, Protein: 2g, Carbs: 36g, Fat: 0g, Fiber: 4g, Sugar: 2g

Chapter 5: AIP Sauces, Condiments and Dressings

Homemade Basil Pesto

Prep Time: 10 minutes
Cooking Time: 0 minutes
Serving Size: 1 cup of pesto

Ingredients

2 cups fresh basil leaves, packed

1/2 cup extra virgin olive oil

1/4 cup coconut cream

2 cloves garlic, minced (optional, omit if sensitive)

1 tablespoon lemon juice

Salt to taste

Cooking Instructions

Clean the basil leaves well and pat dry with paper towels. Put the basil leaves, extra virgin olive oil, coconut cream, minced garlic (if using), and lemon juice in a food processor or blender. Blend until smooth and well combined, scraping down the sides of the bowl as needed. Taste and add salt to taste, blending again to incorporate. Transfer the pesto to a jar or container that fits tightly and refrigerate until needed.

Nutritional Values (per serving - 1 tablespoon):
Calories: 70 kcal, Protein: 1g, Carbs: 1g, Fat: 7g, Fiber: 0g, Sugar: 0g

Coconut Aminos

Prep Time: 5 minutes
Cooking Time: 30-40 minutes
Serving Size: 1 cup

Ingredients

2 cups coconut water

2 tablespoons coconut sugar

1/2 teaspoon sea salt

Cooking Instructions

Coconut water, coconut sugar, and sea salt should all be combined in a small saucepan. The mixture should be brought to a simmer over medium heat, with occasional stirring to dissolve the coconut sugar. After the sugar is dissolved, the heat should be turned down to a low simmer for 30 to 40 minutes, or until the mixture has reduced by half and is syrupy. After turning off the heat and allowing the coconut aminos to cool completely, transfer them to a glass bottle or jar with a tight-fitting lid and keep them in the fridge for up to two weeks.

Nutritional Values (per tablespoon serving):
Calories: 20 kcal, Carbs: 5g, Sugars: 4g

Tahini Dressing

Prep Time: 5 minutes
Serving Size: 4 servings

Ingredients

1/4 cup tahini

2 tablespoons lemon juice

2 tablespoons apple cider vinegar

2 tablespoons extra virgin olive oil

1 clove garlic, minced (optional, omit if sensitive)

2-4 tablespoons water, to thin

Salt to taste

Cooking Instructions

In a small mixing bowl, whisk together tahini, lemon juice, apple cider vinegar, olive oil, and minced garlic (if using). Gradually add water, 1 tablespoon at a time, until the dressing reaches your desired consistency; the amount of water may need to be adjusted depending on how thick your tahini is. Season with salt to taste. Whisk until smooth. Serve over salads, roasted vegetables, or grilled meats.

Nutritional Values (per serving):
Calories: 120 kcal, Protein: 2g, Carbs: 4g, Fat: 11g, Fiber: 1g, Sugar: 0g

Garlic-Herb Aioli

Prep Time: 5 minutes
Serving Size: 1/2 cup of aioli

Ingredients

1/2 cup coconut cream (chilled)

2 tablespoons extra virgin olive oil

1 tablespoon apple cider vinegar

2 cloves garlic, minced (omit if sensitive to garlic)

1 tablespoon chopped fresh herbs (such as parsley, basil, or cilantro)

Salt to taste

Cooking Instructions

In a small mixing bowl, combine the chilled coconut cream, extra virgin olive oil, and apple cider vinegar. Whisk until smooth and well combined. Stir in the minced garlic (if using) and chopped fresh herbs. Season with salt to taste and mix until well combined. Cover and refrigerate the aioli for at least 30 minutes to allow the flavors to meld together. Serve chilled as a dip or spread for meats, veggies, or seafood.

Nutritional Values (per serving 2 tablespoons):
Calories: 120 kcal, Protein: 1g, Carbs: 3g, Fat: 12g, Fiber: 0g, Sugar: 1g

Avocado Lime Dressing

Prep Time: 5 minutes
Serving Size: 6 servings

Ingredients

1 ripe avocado, peeled and pitted

1/4 cup fresh lime juice

2 tablespoons extra virgin olive oil

2 tablespoons chopped fresh cilantro

1 clove garlic, minced (optional, omit if sensitive)

Salt to taste

Water (as needed to adjust consistency)

Cooking Instructions

Combine the avocado, lime juice, olive oil, cilantro, and minced garlic in a blender or food processor. Blend until smooth and creamy. If the dressing is too thick, you can add a little water, one tablespoon at a time, until you reach your desired consistency. Taste and adjust the seasoning with salt as needed. Transfer the dressing to a jar or container with a tight-fitting lid. Store in the refrigerator for up to three to four days.

Nutritional Values (per serving):
Calories: 80 kcal, Protein: 1g, Carbs: 4g, Fat: 7g, Fiber: 3g, Sugar: 0g

Cilantro Lime Chimichurri

Prep Time: 5 minutes
Serving Size: 1 cup

Ingredients

1 cup fresh cilantro, chopped

2 cloves garlic, minced (omit if following strict AIP)

1/4 cup extra virgin olive oil

2 tablespoons lime juice

1/2 teaspoon apple cider vinegar

Salt to taste

Cooking Instructions

Chopped cilantro, minced garlic, extra virgin olive oil, lime juice, and apple cider vinegar should all be combined in a food processor or blender. Pulse until the mixture reaches your desired consistency; it can be blended until smooth or left slightly chunky. Season with salt to taste, adjusting the acidity of the lime juice or vinegar if needed. Transfer the chimichurri to a serving bowl or jar.

Nutritional Values (per serving, based on 2 tablespoons):
Calories: 120 kcal, Protein: 0g, Carbs: 1g, Fat: 14g, Fiber: 0g, Sugar: 0g

Apple Cider Vinaigrette

Prep Time: 5 minutes
Serving Size: 8 servings

Ingredients

1/2 cup apple cider vinegar

1/4 cup extra virgin olive oil

1 tablespoon raw honey (optional, omit if avoiding sweeteners)

1 teaspoon minced garlic

1 teaspoon grated fresh ginger

1/2 teaspoon sea salt

1/4 teaspoon ground black pepper (optional, omit for AIP compliance)

Cooking Instructions

In a small bowl or glass jar, whisk together apple cider vinegar, extra virgin olive oil, raw honey (if using), minced garlic, grated fresh ginger, sea salt, and ground black pepper (if using). Continue whisking until the ingredients are well combined and the vinaigrette is smooth. Taste and adjust seasoning, adding more salt or honey. Serve immediately or store in an airtight container in the refrigerator for up to 1 week. Shake well before serving.

Nutritional Values (per serving):
Calories: 80 kcal, Protein: 0g, Carbs: 2g, Fat: 9g, Fiber: 0g, Sugar: 2g

Carrot Ginger Dressing

Prep Time: 10 minutes
Serving Size: 8 servings

Ingredients

2 medium carrots, peeled and roughly chopped

1-inch piece of fresh ginger, peeled and grated

2 tablespoons apple cider vinegar

2 tablespoons extra virgin olive oil

2 tablespoons water

1 tablespoon coconut aminos

1 tablespoon honey (optional, omit for strict AIP)

Salt to taste

Cooking Instructions

Grated ginger, chopped carrots, apple cider vinegar, olive oil, water, coconut aminos, and honey (if using) should all be combined in a blender or food processor and blended until smooth and well combined. You can adjust the dressing's consistency by adding a little more water if necessary. Taste and adjust the seasoning with salt if necessary. Transfer the dressing to a sealed container and refrigerate for at least 30 minutes to allow the flavors to meld together. Shake well before serving.

Nutritional Values (per serving):
Calories: 35 kcal, Protein: 0.3g, Carbs: 3g, Fat: 2.5g, Fiber: 0.6g, Sugar: 1.6g

Lemon Herb Marinade

Prep Time: 10 minutes
Serving Size: 4

Ingredients

1/4 cup fresh lemon juice

2 tablespoons extra virgin olive oil

2 cloves garlic, minced

1 tablespoon fresh parsley, finely chopped

1 tablespoon fresh thyme leaves, finely chopped

1 tablespoon fresh rosemary, finely chopped

Salt to taste

Cooking Instructions

In a small bowl, whisk together the lemon juice, olive oil, minced garlic, chopped parsley, chopped thyme, and chopped rosemary. Season with salt to taste and mix well to combine.
Use the marinade right away or store it in the refrigerator for up to three days in an airtight container.

Nutritional Values (per serving, marinade only):
Calories: 50 kcal, Protein: 0g, Carbs: 2g, Fat: 5g, Fiber: 0g, Sugar: 0g

Onion Ginger Sauce

Prep Time: 5 minutes
Serving Size: 4 servings

Ingredients

4 green onions, finely chopped

1 tablespoon fresh ginger, grated

2 tablespoons coconut aminos

1 tablespoon apple cider vinegar

1 tablespoon olive oil

1 tablespoon water

Salt to taste

Cooking Instructions

In a small bowl, combine chopped green onions, grated ginger, coconut aminos, apple cider vinegar, olive oil, and water. Stir until well combined. Taste and adjust seasoning with salt if necessary. Let the sauce sit for 10 to 15 minutes to allow the flavors to meld. Serve as a dipping sauce or drizzle over cooked meats, seafood, or vegetables.

Nutritional Values (per serving):
Calories: 35 kcal, Protein: 1g, Carbs: 3g, Fat: 2g, Fiber: 1g, Sugar: 1g

Chapter 6: Drinks and Teas AIP Diet Recipes

Bone Broth

Prep Time: 15 minutes
Cooking Time: 12-24 hours
Serving Size: 8-10 cups

Ingredients

2-3 lbs of grass-fed beef bones or pasture-raised chicken bones

2 carrots, chopped

2 celery stalks, chopped

1 onion, chopped

4 cloves garlic, smashed

2 tablespoons apple cider vinegar

Water, enough to cover the bones

Salt to taste

Cooking Instructions

After preheating the oven to 400°F (200°C), put the bones on a baking sheet and roast them for about 30 minutes, or until they are nicely browned. Then, transfer the roasted bones to a large stockpot or slow cooker, cover the bones completely with water, and add chopped carrots, celery, onion, garlic, and apple cider vinegar. Bring the mixture to a boil over high heat, then reduce the heat to low and let it simmer gently for 12 to 24 hours.

The longer you simmer the mixture, the richer and more flavorful the broth will be. Skim off any foam or impurities that rise to the surface during cooking. After the broth has finished simmering, strain it through a fine mesh sieve or cheesecloth to remove the bones and vegetables, then discard the solids. After allowing the broth to cool, pour it into jars or other storage containers and refrigerate for up to five days. Alternatively, freeze the broth for extended storage.

Nutritional Values (per serving,1 cup):
Calories: 45 kcal, Protein: 5g, Carbs: 2g, Fat: 2g, Fiber: 0g, Sugar: 1g

Peppermint Tea

Prep Time: 1 minute
Cooking Time: 5-7 minutes
Serving Size: 2

Ingredients

1 tablespoon dried peppermint leaves

2 cups water

Cooking Instructions

After bringing two cups of water to a boil in a kettle or saucepan, add the dried peppermint leaves to a teapot or other heat-resistant container, cover the peppermint leaves with boiling water, and let steep for five to seven minutes, allowing the flavor of the peppermint to seep into the water. Finally, strain the tea into cups or mugs.

Ginger Tea

Prep Time: 5 minutes
Cooking Time: 10-15 minutes
Serving Size: 2-4

Ingredients

1-2 inches fresh ginger root, thinly sliced or grated

4 cups filtered water

Optional: Honey (in moderation, if tolerated) or lemon juice for flavor

Cooking Instructions

In a small saucepan, bring the filtered water to a boil. Add the thinly sliced or grated ginger root to the boiling water. Reduce the heat to low and let the ginger simmer in the water for about 10-15 minutes, depending on how strong the flavor you want. Assemble the ginger pieces and strain the tea; pour the ginger tea into mugs and serve hot. You can optionally add a drizzle of honey or a squeeze of lemon juice for extra flavor.

Chamomile Tea

Prep Time: 1 minute
Cooking Time: 5-10 minutes
Serving Size: 1 cup

Ingredients

2 teaspoons dried chamomile flowers

1 cup boiling water

Cooking Instructions

After adding the boiling water to the dried chamomile flowers in a heatproof mug or teapot, cover and steep for five to ten minutes to allow the flavors to infuse. Strain the tea to remove the chamomile flowers.

Dandelion Root Tea

Prep Time: 5 minutes
Cooking Time: 15-20 minutes
Serving Size: 4 cups

Ingredients

2 tablespoons dried dandelion roots (make sure they are harvested from a pesticide-free area)

4 cups water

Cooking Instructions

After washing the dried dandelion roots in cold water to get rid of any dirt or debris, put 4 cups of water in a medium saucepan, add the dried dandelion roots, and boil the water for 10 to 15 minutes. Then, take the saucepan off the heat and let the tea steep for an additional 5 to 10 minutes. Strain the tea to get rid of the dandelion roots, then pour the hot tea into cups

Prep Time: (while water is boiling)
Cooking Time: 5-7 minutes
Serving Size: 2

Ingredients

2 cups water

2-3 rooibos tea bags

Cooking Instructions

In a saucepan, bring two cups of water to a boil. Once boiling, remove from the heat and add the rooibos tea bags. Steep the tea bags in the hot water for five to seven minutes, depending on the strength you want. Then, remove and discard the tea bags and pour the brewed rooibos tea into serving cups.

Coconut Water

Prep Time: 5 minutes
Serving Size: 2 cups of coconut water

Ingredients

1 fresh coconut (green, not mature)

Filtered water

Cooking Instructions

Start by choosing a fresh green coconut, being careful not to choose one that is mature, as mature coconuts have thicker flesh and less water. Use a sturdy knife to carefully chop off the top of the coconut, creating a small opening to access the water inside. Pour the coconut water into a clean glass or container, straining it through a fine mesh sieve if necessary.

Nutritional Values (per serving - 1 cup):
Calories: 45 kcal, Carbs: 9g, Protein: 2g, Fat: 0g, Fiber: 3g Sugar: 6g

Turmeric Latte

Prep Time: 5 minutes
Cooking Time: 5 minutes
Serving Size: 2

Ingredients

2 cups coconut milk (or any other AIP-friendly milk alternative)

1 teaspoon ground turmeric

1/2 teaspoon ground cinnamon

1/4 teaspoon ground ginger

Pinch of ground black pepper (optional, omit if sensitive)

1 tablespoon honey or maple syrup (optional, for sweetness)

Cooking Instructions

Heat the coconut milk in a small saucepan over medium heat, without bringing it to a boil. Whisk in the ground turmeric, ginger, cinnamon, and black pepper. Allow the flavors to mingle for two to three minutes, stirring occasionally. Taste and adjust the sweetness by adding honey or maple syrup, if desired, and stirring until dissolved. Take the mixture off the heat and pour the turmeric latte into mugs.

Nutritional Values (per serving):
Calories: 150 kcal, Protein: 1g, Carbs: 4g, Fat: 14g, Fiber: 1g, Sugar: 3g

Fruit Infused Water

Prep Time: 5 minutes
Infusing Time: 2 hours or overnight
Serving Size: 4

Ingredients

1 liter of filtered water

1 cup of mixed fruits (such as sliced strawberries, sliced oranges, and sliced cucumber)

Cooking Instructions

The mixed fruits should be combined in a large pitcher, then covered and chilled for at least two hours or overnight to allow the flavors to infuse. Serve chilled over ice. Pour filtered water over the fruits and gently stir to combine.

28 DAYS AIP MEAL PLAN

Week 1

- Day 1: AIP Breakfast Skillet

- Day 2: Chicken and Vegetable Stir-Fry

- Day 3: Turmeric Scrambled Eggs

- Day 4: Coconut Berry Bliss Balls

- Day 5: Roasted Sweet Potato and Kale Salad

- Day 6: Stuffed Bell Peppers

- Day 7: Sweet Potato Hash

Week 2

- Day 8: AIP Trail Mix

- Day 9: Cauliflower Rice Stir-Fry

- Day 10: Baked Apples with Cinnamon

- Day 11: Buffalo/Bison

- Day 12: Coconut Flour Pancakes

- Day 13: Portobello Mushroom Burgers

- Day 14: Turmeric Latte

Week 3

- Day 15: AIP Breakfast Burrito Bowl

- Day 16: Grilled Eggplant with Balsamic Glaze

- Day 17: Baked Acorn Squash with Cinnamon

- Day 18: Duck Breast

- Day 19: Coconut Water

- Day 20: Butternut Squash Soup

- Day 21: Lemon Herb Marinade

Week 4

- Day 22: AIP Breakfast Casserole

- Day 23: Cabbage Rolls with Cauliflower Rice

- Day 24: Baked Sweet Potato Chips

- Day 25: Pork Tenderloin

- Day 26: Coconut Aminos

- Day 27: Sweet Potatoes

- Day 28: Apple Cider Vinaigrette

Feel free to shuffle the days or repeat any recipes based on your preferences and nutritional needs.

Recommended Supplements to Support Healing

Although the Autoimmune Protocol (AIP) diet emphasizes whole foods high in nutrients to promote healing and lower inflammation, adding specific supplements can help those who suffer from autoimmune diseases. These supplements can support immune function and improve gut health, among other things.

1 Probiotics

- Role: Probiotics are good bacteria that boost immunity and maintain a balanced microbiome to support gut health.

- Benefits: Supplementing with probiotics has been linked to better digestion, lowered inflammatory levels, and strengthened immune function.

- Recommended Form: Seek out premium probiotic supplements with a range of strains, such as Bifidobacterium and Lactobacillus species.

2. Digestive Enzymes

- Role: In order to promote optimal digestion and nutrient assimilation, digestive enzymes help break down and absorb nutrients from foods.

- Benefits: Digestive enzyme supplements can improve nutrient absorption and reduce digestive discomfort, including gas and bloating, especially in people with impaired gut health.

- Recommended Form: Select a broad-spectrum digestive enzyme supplement that aids in the breakdown of proteins, fats, and carbohydrates by including lipases, amylases, and proteases.

3 Omega-3 Fatty Acids

- Role: The anti-inflammatory qualities of omega-3 fatty acids, especially those of eicosapentaenoic acid (EPA) and docosahexaenoic acid (DHA), promote cardiovascular and mental health.

- Benefits: Omega-3 fatty acid supplements can help lower inflammation, maintain joint health, and enhance mood stability and brain function.

- Recommended Form: To get the bioactive forms of omega-3 fatty acids, EPA and DHA, think about taking supplements made of algae or fish oil.

4 Collagen

- Role: The primary structural protein in the body, collagen is necessary to keep the skin, bones, and connective tissues intact.

- Benefits: Collagen supplements can improve joint function and mobility, support gut health, and encourage skin elasticity and hydration

- Recommended Form: Select hydrolyzed collagen supplements for supporting gut health and tissue repair, as they are highly bioavailable and easily digestible.

5 Vitamin D

- Role: An essential vitamin for immune system function, healthy bones, and general wellbeing is vitamin D

- Benefits: Vitamin D supplements can help the body's defenses against disease, lessen inflammation, and increase the body's ability to absorb calcium and form bones.

- Recommended Form: Rather than taking vitamin D2 supplements, choose vitamin D3 supplements since they are more bioactive and efficient at increasing the body's vitamin D levels.

6 Magnesium

- Role: The body uses magnesium as a necessary mineral for hundreds of enzymatic processes, including the synthesis of energy, the contraction of muscles, and the transmission of nerve signals.

- Benefits: Magnesium supplements can improve sleep quality and relaxation, reduce cramping in the muscles, and control blood pressure and sugar levels

- Recommended Form: Select magnesium malate, glycinate, or citrate for maximum bioavailability and absorption.

7 L-Glutamine

- Role: One amino acid that is essential for preserving the integrity of the intestinal lining and promoting the function of the gut barrier is glutamine.

- Benefits: By reducing intestinal permeability (leaky gut), repairing and healing the gut lining, and easing the symptoms of digestive disorders, L-glutamine supplements can help.

- Recommended Form: To support gut health, look for L-glutamine powder or capsules that are easy to take as a supplement and think about including it in your daily routine.

8 Turmeric/Curcumin

- Role: Curcumin, a strong anti-inflammatory substance with antioxidant qualities that boost immune system performance and lessen inflammation, is found in turmeric

- Benefits: Taking supplements containing turmeric or curcumin can support joint health, ease pain and inflammation brought on by autoimmune diseases, and enhance general wellbeing

- Recommended Form: To improve absorption and bioavailability, choose standardized curcumin supplements that also contain piperine, or black pepper extract.

9 Zinc

- Role: Zinc is a necessary mineral for DNA synthesis, wound healing, and immune system function

- Benefits: Zinc supplements can improve wound healing, lower inflammation, strengthen the immune system, and improve skin health

- Recommended Form: Instead of taking zinc oxide supplements, choose zinc picolinate or zinc citrate, as they are more readily absorbed and have fewer adverse effects on the gastrointestinal tract.

10 Vitamin C

- Role: Strong antioxidant vitamin C promotes tissue repair, collagen synthesis, and immunological function

- Benefits: Taking vitamin C supplements can improve wound healing, lower oxidative stress, strengthen the immune system, and support healthy skin

- Recommended Form: For the best absorption and bioavailability, select vitamin C supplements that contain ascorbic acid, calcium ascorbate, or magnesium ascorbate.

N.B *Choose high-quality supplements from reliable brands to ensure purity, potency, and safety. Keep in mind that supplements are meant to supplement, not replace, a nutrient-rich diet and lifestyle. Think about introducing supplements gradually and monitoring your body's response to ensure tolerability and efficacy.*

Transitioning Off AIP: Reintroduction Phase

You may eventually reach a point where you're ready to reintroduce certain foods back into your diet as you make progress on your AIP journey and notice improvements in your overall health and symptoms. The reintroduction phase gives you the opportunity to determine your specific dietary sensitivity and create a personalized, sustainable eating plan.

1. Reintroduce one food at a time in small amounts, starting with less likely to cause reactions. Observe how your body reacts to the food, both right away and in the hours and days that follow
2. After reintroducing a particular food, note any symptoms or mood swings you experience. Common reactions include headaches, fatigue, joint pain, rashes, and stomach problems.
3. Observe whether a food that has been reintroduced causes symptoms or reactions, record the intensity and duration of any reactions, and decide if it is worth reintroducing the food in the future based on your findings.
4. Focus on developing a customized approach to eating that supports your health and well-being while allowing for flexibility and enjoyment. Based on your findings during the reintroduction phase, modify your diet to exclude or limit foods that cause adverse reactions.

INDEX

Coconut Water 107
Cornish Hen 71
Crispy Baked Plantain Chips 52
Cucumber Avocado Boats 37
Dandelion Root Tea 105
Duck Breast 70
Fruit Infused Water109
Garlic-Herb Aioli 91
Ginger Tea 103
Grilled Eggplant with Balsamic Glaze 59
Homemade Basil Pesto 88
Japanese Sweet Potatoes 82
Lamb Chops 75
Lemon Herb Marinade 96
Mashed Turnips with Herbs 58
Noodles with Pesto 46
Onion Ginger Sauce 97
Peppermint Tea 102
Plantain Waffles 26
Pork Tenderloin 76
Portobello Mushroom Burgers 48
Quail 72
Roasted Sweet Potato and Kale Salad 42
Rooibos Tea 106
Smoked Salmon and Avocado Wrap 24
Spinach and Mushroom Avocado Dressing 61
Stuffed Acorn Squash and Cranberries 63
Stuffed Bell Peppers 49
Sweet Potatoes 81
Sweet Potato Hash 12
Tahini Dressing 90
Turmeric Coconut Porridge 29
Turmeric Scrambled Eggs 20
Turmeric Latte 108
Turkey Thighs 68
Venison 78

White Potatoes 83
Yuca 84
Zucchini Noodles with Pesto 16

REFERENCES

About the Office of Autoimmune Disease Research (OADR-ORWH) | Office of Research on Women's Health. (n.d.). https://orwh.od.nih.gov/OADR-ORWH

Autoimmune Association. (2023, December 16). *Disease Information - Autoimmune Association.* https://autoimmune.org/disease-information/

Christovich, A., & Luo, X. (2022). Gut microbiota, leaky gut, and autoimmune diseases. *Frontiers in Immunology*,

Clinic, C. (2024, March 29). *A little of this and that: Your guide to the AIP diet.* Cleveland Clinic. https://health.clevelandclinic.org/aip-diet-autoimmune-protocol-diet

Konijeti, G. G., Kim, N., Lewis, J. D., Groven, S., Chandrasekaran, A., Grandhe, S., Caroline, D., Singh, E., Oliveira, G., Wang, X., Molparia, B., & Torkamani, A. (2017). Efficacy of the autoimmune protocol diet for inflammatory bowel Disease. *Inflammatory Bowel Diseases*, *23*(11), 2054–2060. https://doi.org/10.1097/mib.0000000000001221

Mailing, L., PhD. (2020, July 5). *The evidence behind the autoimmune protocol diet (and how to try AIP)*. Lucy Mailing, PhD. *Research Breakdown on Autoimmune Protocol (AIP) diet - examine*. (n.d.). https://examine.com/diets/aip-diet/research/

Shaheen, W., Quraishi, M. N., & Iqbal, T. (2022). Gut microbiome and autoimmune disorders. *Clinical and Experimental Immunology (Print)*, *209*(2), 161–174. https://doi.org/10.1093/cei/uxac057

Wu, H., & Wu, E. (2012). The role of gut microbiota in immune homeostasis and autoimmunity. *Gut Microbes*, *3*(1), 4–14. https://doi.org/10.4161/gmic.19320